Managing Epilepsy
A Clinical Handbook

This book is dedicated to my wife and family and especially to our daughter Jane, who, despite having her teenage years disrupted by epilepsy, grew through it all, and emerged a wonderful and talented young woman.

Managing Epilepsy
A Clinical Handbook

Malcolm P. Taylor
MB, ChB, FRCGP
Former General Practitioner
Doncaster

Illustrated by Jane Taylor

Publication of this book was generously supported
by educational grants from:

British Epilepsy Association

The Centre for Community Neurological Studies
Leeds Metropolitan University/NEUROEDUCATION
(York Health NHS Trust)

The RCGP/NSE Educational Fellowship for Epilepsy

Blackwell
Science

© 2000
Published by
Blackwell Science Ltd
Editorial Offices:
Osney Mead, Oxford OX2 0EL
25 John Street, London WC1N 2BS
23 Ainslie Place, Edinburgh EH3 6AJ
350 Main Street, Malden
  MA 02148 5018, USA
54 University Street, Carlton
  Victoria 3053, Australia
10, rue Casimir Delavigne
  75006 Paris, France

Other Editorial Offices:
Blackwell Wissenschafts-Verlag GmbH
Kurfürstendamm 57
10707 Berlin, Germany

Blackwell Science KK
MG Kodenmacho Building
7–10 Kodenmacho Nihombashi
Chuo-ku, Tokyo 104, Japan

First published 2000

Set by
Sparks Computer Solutions Ltd, Oxford
http://www.sparks.co.uk
Printed and bound in Great Britain by
the Alden Press Ltd, Oxford and Northampton

The Blackwell Science logo is a
trade mark of Blackwell Science Ltd,
registered at the United Kingdom
Trade Marks Registry

For further information on
Blackwell Science, visit our website:
www.blackwell-science.com

DISTRIBUTORS

Marston Book Services Ltd
PO Box 269
Abingdon
Oxon OX14 4YN
(*Orders:* Tel: 01235 465500
        Fax: 01235 465555)

USA
Blackwell Science, Inc.
Commerce Place
350 Main Street
Malden, MA 02148 5018
(*Orders:* Tel: 800 759 6102
        781 388 8250
        Fax: 781 388 8255)

Canada
Login Brothers Book Company
324 Saulteaux Crescent
Winnipeg, Manitoba R3J 3T2
(*Orders:* Tel: 204 837-2987
        Fax: 204 837-3116)

Australia
Blackwell Science Pty Ltd
54 University Street
Carlton, Victoria 3053
(*Orders:* Tel: 03 9347 0300
        Fax: 03 9347 5001)

A catalogue record for this title
is available from the British Library

ISBN 0-632-05882-X

Library of Congress
Cataloging-in-Publication data

Taylor, Malcolm P.
  Managing epilepsy: a clinical handbook/
Malcolm P. Taylor; illustrated by Jane
Taylor.—2nd ed.
    p.; cm
  Rev ed. of: Managing epilepsy in primary
care/Maclocm P. Taylor. 1996.
  Includes bibliographical references and
index
ISBN 0-632-05882-X
  1. Epilepsy. 2. Primary care (Medicine)
I. Taylor, Malcolm P. Managing epilepsy in
primary care. II. Title.
  [DNLM: 1. Epilepsy—therapy. 2. Primary
Health Care. WL385 T244m 2000]
  RC372.T39 2000
  616.8'53—dc21
                            00-059904

Contents

Preface, vii

Acknowledgements, ix

1 Epilepsy, Past and Present, 1

2 The Nature of Epilepsy: Aetiology and Epidemiology, 12

3 The Basis for Diagnosis: Recognizing Causes, Seizures and Syndromes, 19

4 Making the Diagnosis: Is it Epilepsy, 33

5 Treatment: General Principles, Anti-Epileptic Drug Therapy, Surgery and Other Treatment, 44

6 Treatment: Individual Anti-Epileptic Drug Profiles, 68

7 Epilepsy and the Individual: Epilepsy in Children and Adolescents, in Women, in Learning Disability and in the Elderly 84

8 Living with Epilepsy: Information, Support and Counselling, 108

9 Living with Epilepsy: 100 Common Questions and Answers, 123

10 Improving Services: a Structure for Care, 147

11 The Role of the Nurse in Epilepsy, 159

Appendix 1: Sources of Help and Advice, 167

Appendix 2: Managing Epilepsy in General Practice: Audit, 172

Appendix 3: Purchasing and Providing Epilepsy Outpatient Services: A Guide to Good Practice, 177

Appendix 4: Community Nurse Learning Disability Assessment of Epilepsy, 186

References and Recommended Further Reading, 193

Index, 199

Preface

This book's predecessor *Managing Epilepsy in Primary Care* was, as its title implied, aimed at UK general practice. Despite having a title that appeared to limit its appeal, and some content specific to primary care, it found a wider audience. The general sections on diagnosis, anti-epileptic drug therapy, other treatments, general management, and patient information and support were found useful in secondary care as well as primary care, by nurses (and specialist nurses in particular), in learning disability, by teachers, and by some patients and families. To recognize and encourage this wider readership the new edition has a change of title.

The main content and presentation remain unchanged apart from being brought up to date. The sections on treatment include details of new anti-epileptic drugs, and an account of the emerging roles of the drugs that were new or recent at the time of the previous edition. The section in Chapter 7 on 'Epilepsy in women' has been expanded, and a new section on 'Epilepsy and learning disability' fills an obvious gap. There is an entirely new chapter, 'The Role of the Nurse in Epilepsy', needed because the epilepsy specialist nurse is now recognized as a crucial member of any epilepsy service, and practice nurses and other nurses are taking an increasing part in epilepsy care.

It is still intended to be a 'How to do it book' rather than a textbook. I hope that it helps the reader to approach epilepsy care in a practical, caring and effective way.

MALCOLM TAYLOR

Acknowledgements

This further edition owes everything to the support of Henry Smithson, Brian Chappell and Mike Moran. Without their enthusiasm for the first edition, and their persistence in securing a successor, it simply would not have happened. The British Epilepsy Association provided invaluable support again, and I thank Monica Cooper and her colleagues for vetting and adding to the chapters on information, common questions and sources of help. Thank you too to Danielle Luxford and her colleagues in the Benefits Agency for putting me straight on benefit issues. To Velma Boulter, Carole Doran, Pippa Roberts and Keith Redhead for their helpful comments on the new chapter. 'The Role of the Nurse in Epilepsy'. To Mike Kerr, Jacqui Brewster, Tracy Lumb, Heather Gregory and Helen Wilkinson for the considerable help they gave in drafting the section on 'Epilepsy and learning disability'. And finally, grateful thanks to my editor John Ashworth, whose guidance (and emails) made the rewriting surprisingly swift and easy.

MALCOLM TAYLOR

Epilepsy, Past and Present 1

Why begin by referring to the past in a practical 'How to do it' book for today? The reason is that **how we provide care for patients with epilepsy today and how patients and families are affected by it are both uniquely tied up with the history of epilepsy**. Many of the prejudices and difficulties which patients with epilepsy still meet within society today have their roots in folk tradition. Current medical practice, and the distribution of specialist epilepsy services in the UK, also have their roots in the medical profession's own historical perceptions of epilepsy and commitment to its care. A knowledge and understanding of this background can be helpful when providing care for individuals, and indispensable for those involved in arguing and negotiating for improved specialist services.

This chapter sets out to explain: why patients sometimes feel the way they do; why services are so inadequate; how things are changing in response to new technology, new drugs and pressure from patients and part of the profession; the contribution of general practice to the changes; and the emerging challenges to general practice.

The distant past

A convulsive seizure is quite disturbing to witness, capable of provoking awe, dismay and even disgust. In earlier times this understandably made epilepsy an object of superstitious belief. Hippocrates was the first to attribute the origin of convulsive disorders to the brain in his discourse *On the Sacred Diseases*, around 450 BC. Despite this, the notion that the person with epilepsy was 'possessed' persisted, and New Testament stories attested to this belief. The story in the Gospel of St Mark (9.16–29) about 'the healing of the boy with an evil spirit' provides a vivid picture of the effects of having epilepsy on a child, and a detailed description of a tonic–clonic seizure and its after-effects (Fig. 1.1): 'Teacher, I brought you my son, who is possessed by a spirit that has robbed him of speech. Whenever it seizes him, it throws him to the ground. He foams at the mouth, gnashes his teeth and becomes rigid ... When the spirit saw Jesus, it immediately

1

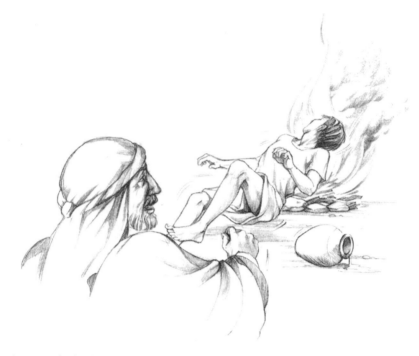

Fig. 1.1 'The healing of the boy with an evil spirit' (Gospel of St Mark, 9.16–29).

threw the boy into a convulsion. He fell to the ground and rolled around, foaming at the mouth ... From childhood, ... it has often thrown him into the fire or water to kill him.' The same story in St Matthew's Gospel refers to the boy as an 'epileptic'. Even today, the term 'epileptic', when used as a noun, suggests that an individual is not normal, is somehow different, perhaps 'not right in the head'. Not surprisingly, sufferers prefer to be described as 'people with epilepsy', a convention which will be followed in this book. The term 'epilepsy' itself derives from the Greek *epi lambamo*, which means 'a taking hold of, to seize, or to possess'.

The recent past: nineteenth century onwards

Developments in understanding

Modern understanding of the nature of epilepsy began in the middle of the nineteenth century. It was then recognized that epilepsy was not just one disorder, but a symptom which had many manifestations and causes. One of the most important contributors to this understanding was Dr Hughlings

Jackson (1835–1911), who is particularly remembered for describing focal motor epilepsy, which is named after him, and which he observed in his wife. His definition of epilepsy still remains as good as any today: '**A convulsion is but a symptom, and implies only that there is an occasional, an excessive and a disorderly discharge of nerve tissue**' [1]. French descriptions of seizures have left us a legacy of terms still used today, such as grand mal, petit mal, absence and déjà vu.

Twentieth-century advances in diagnostic techniques, starting with radiology and electroencephalography, and, more recently, computer scanning, magnetic resonance imaging and isotope scanning, have made it increasingly possible to identify underlying causes. The nature of seizure activity is now better understood and classified, and it has become possible to identify specific epilepsy syndromes, with implications for treatment and prognosis.

Developments in treatment

Although understanding increased, no effective treatment existed until the bromides were introduced in 1857. Potassium bromide, which was known to cause temporary impotence in men, was first used to treat epilepsy in the belief that sexual excess and masturbation caused fits. As it turned out, potassium bromide actually worked in controlling seizures, but the first really important advance was the introduction of phenobarbitone in 1912, followed by phenytoin in 1938. In 1945 the first of the succinimides brought a major advance in the treatment of petit mal. For many years, phenobarbitone and phenytoin were the mainstay of treatment. They were often given together, and sometimes with other drugs; consequently, sedation and drug intoxication were serious problems. Following phenobarbitone and phenytoin, the next important arrivals were carbamazepine and sodium valproate. The former, although around for some years, was not used much until the early 1970s, and sodium valproate was first used in the UK in 1973.

When serum drug level measurements became available in the 1970s, it was found that drugs could be used more precisely, more effectively and often singly. Polytherapy gave way to monotherapy, but not completely. Some patients still needed more than one drug for control, but the benefits to many patients in terms of fewer seizures and reduced side-effects have been remarkable.

Because they are both effective, and both have fewer side-effects than phenobarbitone or phenytoin, sodium valproate and carbamazepine have emerged as the main first-line drugs and remain so despite the arrival of newer drugs. The development of new anti-epileptic drugs remained static for over a decade until 1989 when vigabatrin was licensed. Since then there has been a stream of new drugs: lamotrigine (1991), gabapentin (1993), topiramate (1995), tiagabine (1998), and more recently piracetam (for myoclonus only), oxcarbazepine (2000), and levetiracetam which is expected to be licensed shortly. Initially used as add-on drugs, the new arrivals are already finding their places. They appear to vary in effectiveness, some have been found to have specific effects in certain types of epilepsy, some are remarkably free from side-effects, and others—some of the more potent—have more side-effects.

What are the implications of this plethora of choice for the GP or other non-epilepsy specialist? At first sight, the task seems to be getting more complicated, more and more a job for specialists. Some of the newer drugs, especially topiramate, though effective, are tricky to use, have a lot of side-effects and are clearly for specialist use. Evidence is emerging that vigabatrin is responsible for more cases of visual field defect than was previously realized, and this requires frequent monitoring. Gabapentin, on the other hand, though a less effective drug, is straightforward to use, has few side-effects and is suitable for GP use. In the end, the important point to bear in mind is that **for most patients with epilepsy, at present, the effective use of the present first-line anti-epileptic drugs remains the mainstay of treatment**. This is something the GP or other non-epilepsy specialist can do.

Developments in services

In the nineteenth century, people with severe epilepsy were often confined in lunatic asylums, despite having no mental disorder. Towards the end of the century, a more enlightened approach led to the establishment of 'epilepsy colonies', based on an earlier colony in Bielefeld, Germany. The colonies were small self-contained communities where those with severe epilepsy were able to live and work in a sheltered environment. Although an enlightened movement, its effect was to segregate, and even separate by sex, large numbers of people who were normal apart from having seizures.

Specialist medical interest in epilepsy in the nineteenth century was limited and mainly concentrated in London, notably at the National Hospital for the Paralysed and Epileptic (now The National Hospital), where that great authority on epilepsy, Sir William Gowers, was physician. Neurology, as a speciality, has remained small, particularly when compared with other developed countries. Even in 1950, two years after the inception of the National Health Service (NHS), there were only 49 consultant posts in neurology, and these were mainly in London and the South-East. Then, as now, few neurologists had a particular interest in epilepsy.

The last 45 years

Our present specialist services for epilepsy have developed mainly from their earlier roots in neurology and psychiatry, to be joined in recent times by clinical pharmacology. The medical specialities now involved in the treatment of epilepsy include neurology, neuropsychiatry, clinical pharmacology, neurosurgery, neurophysiology, general medicine and paediatrics.

The current surge of interest in epilepsy, among specialists and GPs, is due in part to the arrival of new and effective anti-epileptic drugs, and improved opportunities for surgical cure linked to advances in imaging technology. These, added to our greater understanding of epilepsy and ability to use existing drugs more effectively, provide an exciting prospect. However, for patients to benefit, adequate services are needed both in general practice and from specialists, and specialist services specifically for epilepsy are scarce. Fortunately, where such services exist, the quality is high, and they provide good models for the future development of services.

Working party recommendations for epilepsy services

There have been recommendations galore for improving and developing services in a succession of government-sponsored reports over the past 45 years or so [2–5]. Of particular interest was the *Report of the Working Group on Services for People with Epilepsy* [5]. This reported in 1984 and finally published its findings in 1986. It reviewed and added to the recommendations of earlier reports, and listed among its criticisms of hospital services, 'long delays in obtaining appointments, inadequate or irregular follow-up and supervision, lack of continuity of care, and lack of attention to social requirements or counselling'. Among its recommendations were detailed requirements for district clinics, including the need for a member of staff to foster links with other health service facilities and other organizations—a role later taken on with great effect by the first epilepsy specialist liaison nurses. GPs were expected to be responsible for the initial recognition and referral of patients with suspected epilepsy. District hospitals were to manage diagnosis and investigation, returning patients to general practitioners for follow-up. Patients whose seizures were difficult to control or required particular expertise were to be referred to tertiary centres. The response to this report and to its predecessors was disappointing. Underlying this had been a low priority given to epilepsy services within the NHS, plus a chronic shortfall in the numbers of specialist neurologists in the UK, especially any with a particular interest in epilepsy. In the early 1990s, there were only 21 clinics in the UK specifically for epilepsy and seven special centres [6]. The Netherlands had, in comparison, 10 times the number of neurologists for an equivalent population.

The 1990s has seen renewed interest and activity in developing epilepsy services, with a succession of reports identifying needs and making recommendations for services. The first of these recent contributions to the debate on services was a report written in 1993 by a group of clinicians involved in epilepsy services including GPs. It was published as 'An Epilepsy Needs Document' [7] with the approval of the Joint Epilepsy Council representing all major patient organizations and care providers. This document described services for epilepsy in the UK as 'poor in quality, fragmentary and poorly organized'. It set out to define and quantify the scope, content and standards of medical, paramedical and nursing services required in primary care and from specialist centres, with the intention of influencing purchasers and providers. This report was followed by 'Epilepsy needs revisited' in 1998 [8]. The Epilepsy Task Force, a grouping of professionals and representatives from consumer bodies, first produced a guide to purchasing and providing epilepsy outpatient services (see Appendix 3) and later, in 1999, went on to produce the *Epilepsy Task Force Service Development Kit* [9]. The same year saw another 'tool kit' *Epilepsy Care— Making it Happen* [10], and a major report by the Clinical Standards Advisory Group (CSAG) *Services for Patients with Epilepsy* [11]. It seems that there is no shortage of excellent advice and guidance for those wishing to improve epilepsy services—it merely requires the will and the resources. Interestingly, the British Epilepsy Association's (BEA) comment on the government response to the prestigious CSAG report was to describe it as 'lukewarm', and to ask 'is this a new age for epilepsy, or just another false dawn?'

Progress may be slow, but progress there is. At the end of the decade the number of specialist epilepsy clinics in the UK was 127 according to CSAG, and 100 (60 adult, 40 children) according to the BEA. Epilepsy specialist nurses are seen as key to services and there are now about 100.

Changes in the management of epilepsy in primary care

Many GPs perceive difficulties

It has been shown that it is possible to improve care, in terms of seizure control and reduced drug side-effects, in general practice [12,13] as well as in hospital studies [14,15]. But it is not seen by GPs as easy to do. Of Doncaster practitioners replying to a survey in 1987, two-thirds, while acknowledging responsibility for the overall care of patients with epilepsy, reported difficulties in diagnosis, counselling and especially in the use of drugs. The problem lies in part in the numbers; an individual practitioner will only have about 10–15 patients with established epilepsy altogether, two or three of these with difficult-to-control epilepsy, and is likely to see only one or two new cases each year. This may not be many to look after but provides little basis to acquire or retain expertise.

Audit—identifying deficiencies in care

Despite epilepsy being seen as difficult, there is a steady increase in interest in it in UK general practice. Much of this interest has evolved around audit, for which epilepsy has provided an ideal topic, offering small numbers of patients and clear criteria. At any rate, surveys and audits of epilepsy care carried out in general practice have helped to identify overall deficiencies in care [16–21] (including those involving specialist services as well as general practice). These findings have included: 'poor seizure control, inadequate follow-up, ineffective use of drugs and lack of advice and information'. Misdiagnosis has been identified as a serious problem, involving 26% of patients referred to special centres with a diagnosis of epilepsy [22], and 23.8% in a specialist review in general practice [23]. Common causes of difficulty are non-epileptic seizures (pseudo-seizures), partial seizures being missed and syncope misdiagnosed as epilepsy.

The catalogue of apparent deficiencies in care revealed by audit should not obscure its positive consequences. Practices involved in audit have gone on not only to improve what they do for their own patients, but also to influence developments in specialist services as well as the rest of general practice. Audits in a Doncaster practice acted as a spur to the development of a district service incorporating a specialist clinic, guidelines for shared care and have pioneered a community-based epilepsy specialist liaison nursing service [24]. Hall and Ross [20], after reporting on audit in his own practice, went on to develop audit material for general use in collaboration with the British Epilepsy Association.

Epilepsy research and general practice

Also on the positive side is the contribution of UK general practice to epilepsy research, particularly into its epidemiology and natural history. This has been aided by the structure of primary care in the UK, which allows a comprehensive and unselected view of a disorder such as epilepsy, by allowing full case identification and follow-up when patients move. The pioneering work of Crombie et al. [25], and of Pond et al. [26], has been succeeded more recently by the National General Practice Study of Epilepsy (NGPSE) [27]. This large prospective study of newly diagnosed epilepsy started in 1984 and involves 275 GPs and 1195 patients. This study has already added to our understanding of prognosis [28,29], the frequency of seizure types [30], the relevance of syndromic classification to general practice [31], the social and psychological effects of a recent diagnosis of epilepsy [32] and the cost of epilepsy [33].

The need for guidance

The contribution of general practice requires definition, and *Epilepsy: a general practice problem*, published by the Royal College of General Practitioners (RCGP) [34], goes some way to meeting this need. This document is concerned with educational needs, the interface with secondary care, guidelines for management and service development. Other information about how to actually clinically manage epilepsy in general practice has to be derived from specialist texts, local guidelines specifically developed for shared care, including primary care, such as those in Cumbria, Leeds, Ireland and Doncaster, and of course this book.

The consequences of having epilepsy

Epilepsy carries unique burdens and consequences for patients and families. Even today, in addition to having to cope with seizures, those affected complain of feeling 'different' or stigmatized. Some may have an associated disability, such as learning disability. Certainly, many face significant problems in social life and in employment.

A thirst for information

There is no shortage of evidence about what patients lack or feel that they want. Lloyd Jones, in her illuminating trainee audit in 1980 [16], observed that: 'patients were not being counselled sufficiently on the problems of epilepsy', and that 'over half the patients considered themselves to be unacceptable to the rest of society'. A British Epilepsy Association survey in 1991 [35] found that 'respondents would like an increase in provision of services and in the information conveyed', concern was expressed about 'the extent of management and of experimentation left to the patient and care giver'. Dawkins *et al.*, in a general practice study [36], found that patients know little more than the general population about epilepsy. Of patients attending a Belfast hospital clinic in 1993 [37], 90% wanted more information about the disease, three-quarters felt they had not been given enough information about drug side-effects and over 60% wanted to talk to someone other than the consultant, with a preference for a specialist nurse. A pilot study in 1993 [38] for a 'Quality of Life and Care in Epilepsy' survey in the Mersey region, combined with an audit of primary care involving 40 practices, found that, although two-thirds of patients saw their GP as primarily responsible for their care, only 60% felt it was easy to talk to the GP about their epilepsy, and around one-third of adult patients and one-quarter of parents considered that they had not been given enough information. When the place of personal continuity of care in general practice, in allowing discussion of personally important aspects of having epilepsy, is explored [39], seeing the same doctor emerges as being less important than improving doctors' communication skills and paying specific attention to the psychosocial aspects of epilepsy as well as to seizure control.

A clear picture emerges of a group of people and their families who continue to feel different and disadvantaged, who are lacking in information and support and whose wider needs are ignored. A great deal has been done in providing help and information, as well as lobbying for improved services by the various epilepsy associations, but much more is needed, at hospital, practice and community levels. Recently [24], specialist epilepsy nurses, some community-based, have been shown to be very effective in not only improving epilepsy control but in meeting these very important wider needs, in patients' homes, schools and residential homes.

What next? A challenge to primary care

Purchasing services

The development of services for those with epilepsy has, in general, failed to match the potential demonstrated in the few specialist centres, or the expectations of those affected by epilepsy. The scanty provision of specialist services has a historical basis and, although there is a definite movement and interest in increasing services, it could, given the shortfall in consultant neurologist numbers, take a long time to be redressed. However, general practice can now help speed the process. UK general practice in the 1990s was able to influence the development of services as never before, in the direct purchasing of services through 'fundholding', and in advising purchaser health authorities through 'commissioning'. More recently (1999), the creation of Primary Care Groups (PCGs), consisting of larger groupings of general practices, increases this potential. The opportunity presented by this novel situation to improve epilepsy services should be seized. This is explored in Chapter 10.

Improving practice-based care

Most patients with epilepsy are registered with a GP, who has to cope whatever the state of specialist support available to his or her patients. Most GPs accept some sort of role in epilepsy management, although a minority regard it as totally a job for specialists. An increasing number of practices have undertaken audit of their epilepsy care, and through this are developing interest in epilepsy and in improving services. In a few, that interest has extended to developing competence in diagnosis, changing and adjusting medication and providing advice and support. Some practice nurses, increasingly competent in the chronic disease management of diabetes and asthma, are taking an interest in epilepsy, particularly where influenced by the growing band of specialist nurses. They are finding patients and families eager and grateful for information, support and counselling. This should come as no surprise, for after all, most of the problems identified by patients are to do with the consequences of having epilepsy.

Even where specialist epilepsy services are available, the primary care contribution to achieving an accurate diagnosis in newly presenting patients, to adjusting treatment in established patients, and to providing long-term support, is essential for good care. The CSAG *Services for Patients with Epilepsy* report [11] recommends the appointment of a lead GP within a group practice to take lead responsibility for improving epilepsy services, but it is not quite clear what this involves. If it means not simply negotiating improved secondary care services, but the establishment of a practice-based system of chronic disease management for epilepsy similar to that for asthma and diabetes, which the document also explores, then similar funding would be needed. Epilepsy care in general practice deserves encouragement. In a modern NHS, led by *Health of the Nation* targets and payments directed at chronic disease management in primary care, the inclusion of epilepsy would help. In the end, of course, it is up to the individual doctor to decide how much he or she can contribute to either getting specialist services improved, or to improving the care within the practice.

2 The Nature of Epilepsy: Aetiology and Epidemiology

Patients and relatives naturally want to know what epilepsy is and what the implications of having it are. They want to know what is causing it, whether it is serious, especially whether it is a risk to life, whether it is due to a tumour or brain haemorrhage, if it can it be cured and how it will affect life. They complain about the lack of information provided by doctors and suspect that doctors do not always know. For their part, doctors need to know not only what to tell individual patients, but also the extent and nature of the overall task facing them in providing services.

In general, patients and relatives can be given an encouraging prospect (Fig. 2.1). Serious causes of epilepsy, such as cerebral tumour, are rare and the traditional view that the prognosis of treated epilepsy is poor, based on hospital and institutional studies, has been shown to be mistaken. Of course, it is important to attempt to define the underlying cause for each patient, especially one which might be dangerous in its own right. However, in most cases, although a focus of epileptic activity might be inferred, the precise pathology may not be known. Modern imaging, particularly magnetic resonance imaging (MRI), is increasing the pick-up of detectable lesions.

Definitions

So what is epilepsy? Hughlings Jackson put it well enough [1], when he described a seizure as a 'symptom'. **Epilepsy is itself 'a chronic disorder characterized by recurrent unprovoked seizures'.** Usually this is taken to be at least two or more seizures.

Since epilepsy is a recurring symptom, rather than a specific condition, and the underlying cause is often obscure, the study of epilepsy has largely focused on defining and classifying seizures. Classifications of seizures and epilepsy syndromes, and their relevance to management, are dealt with fully in Chapter 3, but it is helpful to recognize that there are two main groups of seizures: **generalized seizures** in which epileptic discharges involve both hemispheres simultaneously from the onset and **partial seizures** in which

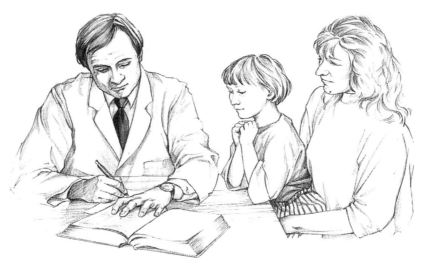

Fig. 2.1 Patients benefit from an opportunity to have questions answered.

epileptic activity starts in a focal area of the brain, where it may remain confined or may spread to be secondarily generalized. Generalized seizures are more common in childhood and partial seizures increasingly common from early adult life onwards as structural causes become more common. A proportion of seizures remain **unclassifiable seizures**.

Where epilepsy develops as a **chronic** phenomenon in relationship to a persisting lesion, nowadays it is often referred to as **remote symptomatic epilepsy**. This helps to differentiate it from seizures which may occasionally be **acute** in response to metabolic or systemic disturbance, and are described as **acute symptomatic seizures**. Acute symptomatic seizures comprised 15% of first seizures in the National General Practice Study of Epilepsy (NGPSE) studies, with alcohol abuse at 6% of the total by far the commonest cause. Drugs commonly causing acute symptomatic seizures include penicillin, isoniazid, hypoglycaemic drugs, psychotropic drugs, bronchodilators and lignocaine.

Metabolic causes of acute symptomatic seizures include pyrexia, hypoglycaemia, electrolyte disturbance, hypoxia, severe myxoedema, hepatic failure and renal failure. (This topic is fully covered by Chadwick [40].)

Aetiology

The possible causes of epilepsy are numerous, and include genetic causes, congenital malformations, infections, tumours, vascular disease and severe head injury. In fact, virtually any cerebral pathology (Fig. 2.2). Nevertheless, in practice, no specific cause can be found in 60–70% of cases, though this seems to be changing since the advent of MRI. In the NGPSE study of newly diagnosed epileptic seizures, the commonest remote symptomatic causes were vascular disease (15%) and tumour (6%). In patients over 60 years of age, cerebrovascular disease accounted for 49% of cases. Tumour was rare under the age of 30 years, but reached 19% between 50 and 59 years.

Epidemiology

Incidence and prevalence

From community studies [41,42], the annual incidence of non-febrile single seizures is 20 per 100 000 and the incidence of new cases of epilepsy is 50 per 100 000. Estimates of the overall risk of an individual having a non-febrile seizure at some time in life is surprisingly high at between 2 and 5%. The

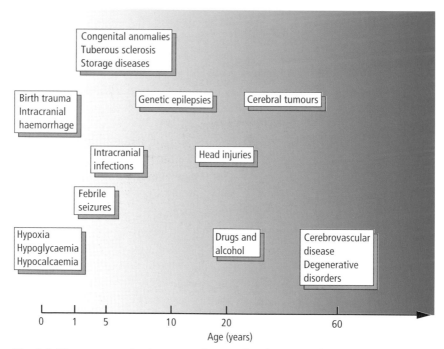

Fig. 2.2 The pattern of seizure aetiology with relation to the age of onset. From Chadwick, D., Cartlidge, N. and Bates, D. *Medical Neurology*. Edinburgh: Churchill Livingstone, 1989.

prevalence of active epilepsy is about 5 per 1000, and it is apparent from the discrepancy between the cumulative lifetime incidence and prevalence, that most patients who develop epilepsy only have it temporarily (Fig. 2.3). Translated to general practice, this means that an individual GP, with a list of about 2000 patients, can expect to have between 10 and 15 patients with active epilepsy on his or her list, and to see one or two new cases each year.

Incidence varies considerably with age. Over three-quarters of patients with epilepsy start with seizures before the age of 18 years, and one-quarter of patients with newly diagnosed epilepsy are under the age of 15 years. Happily, many of the epilepsies of childhood are benign and do not persist into adult life. Rates are lowest in early adult life but rise again in the elderly, who, contrary to general belief, have a high incidence of epilepsy. In the NGPSE study, 24% of new diagnoses were in patients over 60 years, usually in association with cerebrovascular disease and stroke. Since the proportion of elderly in the population is rising, a future increase in elderly patients with epilepsy can be expected.

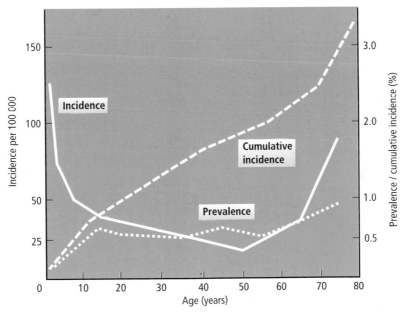

Fig. 2.3 Age-specific cumulative incidence and prevalence rates in Rochester, Minnesota, 1935–74. From Hauser, W.A., Annergers, J.F. and Anderson, V.E. Epidemiology and genetics of epilepsy. In: Ward, A.A., Penry, J.K. and Purpura, D. *Epilepsy*. New York: Raven Press, 1983: 274.

Prevalence and frequency of seizure types

Partial seizures, that is complex partial and secondarily generalized seizures, account for 60% of prevalent cases. Primary generalized tonic–clonic seizures account for about 30% and generalized absence and myoclonus for less than 5%. The incidence of presenting seizures, in new cases in the NGPSE study, was a secondarily generalized seizure in 36%, a primary generalized tonic–clonic seizure in 33%, a complex partial seizure in 16%, a simple partial seizure in 4%, an absence seizure in 1% and myoclonus in 1%.

Severity in the population

The range of severity of epilepsy and its associated disabilities in the population is not exactly known. The 'Epilepsy Needs Document' [7] suggests that about one-third of patients have less than one seizure each year, one-third between one and twelve seizures a year and one-third more than one seizure each month (and one-fifth more than one seizure each week). Audits in 26 Doncaster general practices [43] of patients with active epilepsy or on anti-epileptic medication for past epileptic seizures, give figures of 40% seizure-free, 25% with less than one seizure each month and 35% with more than one seizure each month.

The course of epilepsy

For many, epilepsy is fortunately a mild, short-lasting experience. Although recurrence after a first seizure is very common (78% in the NGPSE study), in most cases the total number of seizures is small and the epilepsy short lived, and most of those entering remission do so early. Recent results from the NGPSE study [27] show that 9 years after the index seizure, 86% of patients with definite epilepsy had remissions of 3 years and 68% a remission of 5 years.

In a community survey of 465 patients in Rochester, Minnesota [41], 50% had been in remission for 5 years, 20 years after diagnosis, and were off treatment. A further 20% were in remission and on treatment. In a similar study in Tonbridge (UK) [42], 15 years after diagnosis, only 19% had had a seizure in the previous 2 years and 65% had epilepsy lasting less than 5 years.

The outcome for seizure control in most patients is good.

Prognostic factors

A good prognosis is associated with: seizures precipitated by alcohol, drugs or metabolic disturbances; benign syndromes; or adult-onset idiopathic seizures. A poor prognosis is likely where there is evidence of diffuse cerebral disorder (intellectual or behavioural disturbance); onset of seizures in the first year of life, severe epilepsy syndromes or progressive neurological disorders. Seizure type is of major importance in determining outcome [40]. Remission rates range from 60 to 80% for tonic–clonic seizures alone, to between 20 and 60% for patients with complex partial seizures. The combination of complex partial and secondarily generalized tonic–clonic seizures has a poorer prognosis, but is better if seizures started before the age of 20 years. Overall, childhood epilepsy is more likely to remit than adult-onset epilepsy.

Mortality

That patients with epilepsy have a higher death rate than the non-epileptic population is known from past studies, but few of these have been population-based studies such as the NGPSE study of newly diagnosed epilepsy. Increased mortality has been associated with that due to the underlying cause (e.g. tumour, stroke), to seizure-related causes (e.g. status epilepticus) and to injury. A number of deaths are ascribed to 'sudden unexplained death in epilepsy' (SUDEP) and an increased risk of suicide.

The NGPSE study confirmed increased mortality, with a standardized mortality ratio (SMR) of 3.0 for 'definite epilepsy' and 2.5 for 'definite epilepsy' plus 'possible epilepsy'. Deaths were highest in the first year and were associated with stroke and tumour, which is no surprise. However, even for 'idiopathic cases', the SMR was still increased at 1.6. There were only two seizure-related deaths, one possible suicide and no sudden unexplained deaths.

A prospective survey of deaths in a population in Nova Scotia [44] found that deaths resulting from seizures were 2.68 per 100 000.

Newly diagnosed patients without serious underlying pathology can reasonably be reassured that, although there is a risk of premature death, it is quite small.

Conclusions

The overall picture of epilepsy in the population is one in which many who develop epilepsy remit early, most patients are well controlled, and a minority have frequent, even daily, seizures. Serious underlying causes such as cerebral tumour are uncommon, although more common in the elderly. Common in childhood, epilepsy is becoming increasingly common in old age. Most people with epilepsy are otherwise intellectually quite normal, but in some, it is associated with severe learning disability (25–30% of people with learning disability have epilepsy).

How much epilepsy in a practice?

An average group practice of four doctors will have 40–60 patients with active epilepsy and/or on anti-epileptic medication, and four to six newly diagnosed cases each year. This will include six or seven with learning disability, and perhaps one or two patients with one of the relatively rare epilepsy syndromes of childhood. About 40% of patients are likely to be seizure-free, 35% will have frequent seizures (more than one per month) and the rest will have seizures ranging from one to twelve a year. Many of those with infrequent seizures may be helped by simple advice and intervention. Most patients, seizure-free or not, will benefit from an opportunity to ask questions and have them answered. Overall, it is likely that a review of diagnosis and medication in those with epilepsy in an average practice will reveal opportunities to improve seizure control and reduce the burden of drug side-effects.

The Basis for Diagnosis: Recognizing Causes, Seizures and Syndromes   3

This chapter discusses the need to consider diagnosis at three levels: the underlying cause, seizure type, and where possible, the epilepsy syndrome. Seizure classification is dealt with in detail, but only the more common epilepsy syndromes relevant to general practice are outlined.

Bewildering concepts?

It is no wonder that most doctors and nurses seem to find epilepsy bewildering. To start with, an epileptic seizure is 'but a symptom', with many possible causes (seemingly any cerebral pathology). Next it is classified into many seizure types, the names of which have changed, although not everyone involved seems to recognize this. Terms like 'grand mal' and 'petit mal', which many of us were taught, are no longer used by epilepsy specialists. A new and more practical classification based on whether a seizure is 'generalized' in nature or 'partial' and arising from a 'focus' is becoming standard. Finally, there are also 'epilepsy syndromes'—yet another classification. (An 'epilepsy syndrome' is a cluster of signs and other factors customarily occurring together, e.g. seizure type, aetiology, age of onset, electroencephalogram (EEG) findings.)

Epileptologists consider 'epilepsy syndromes', otherwise known as 'the epilepsies', to be very important, which of course they are, particularly in specialist practice. But the relevance of the current classification to the population of patients with epilepsy seen in general practice has been shown, by the National General Practice Study of Epilepsy (NGPSE) study [31], to be limited. The classification was devised before modern imaging techniques became so effective, and so, for example, what appears clinically to be a generalized seizure, and therefore generalized epilepsy, may, with magnetic resonance imaging (MRI), be shown to be of focal origin, i.e. a partial epilepsy. Despite the shortcomings of the syndrome classification, it is important to recognize its usefulness in understanding and managing some patients, especially those with epilepsy starting in childhood.

Three levels of diagnosis

Causes, seizure type and syndrome together amount to three levels of diagnosis. All of which seems rather a lot to have to grasp for a GP seeing only one or two new cases each year, and with perhaps only 10–15 patients with epilepsy altogether. Is it really useful and if it is, how useful?

In principle, considering diagnosis at the three levels is sensible. An underlying cause may require attention in its own right, for example a cerebral tumour (rare but important) and its resection may lead to the alleviation of the epilepsy. Correct seizure classification is needed to ensure the correct anti-epileptic treatment (actually, it may not matter for most patients, but when it matters, it *really* matters). Finally, making a syndrome diagnosis, where it is possible, may help to predict the likely course and prognosis of an individual patient's epilepsy.

Fortunately, as far as primary care is concerned, common things occur commonly, and rare things only occur often enough to make life interesting. About 60–70% of all cases have no clearly identifiable cause, few causes require treatment in their own right, and most patients with epilepsy in an individual general practice will fall into a small number of seizure types and syndromes.

Although an underlying cause cannot always be demonstrated by 'tests' such as EEGs, computed tomography (CT) and MRI scans, it can often, together with the seizure diagnosis, be inferred from the medical history alone. Important in addition to seizure descriptions are the age of onset of the epilepsy, perinatal history and development, prolonged febrile convulsions, severe head injury, central nervous system (CNS) infection, family history of epilepsy, CNS symptoms and signs.

Practical points

The following should be noted:
• It is important to look for underlying causes, and exclude anything serious in its own right;
• The modern seizure classification into 'generalized' and 'partial' seizures is practical and useful in general practice;
• There are limitations to applying 'syndrome' classification in general practice, but it is useful and important to recognize a small number;
• In most cases the patient's history, particularly a detailed seizure description, will provide the seizure classification, indicate the aetiology and often the syndrome.

Seizure classification

Most doctors and nurses enter practice with little experience of epilepsy and may have witnessed few, if any, seizures ever. In training, we learn about 'grand mal' and 'petit mal' seizures, conveying an idea of fits being 'big and bad' or 'small and not so bad'; 'idiopathic' when the cause is mysterious; and special categories such as 'Jacksonian fits', and 'temporal lobe seizures' with auras and strange behaviour.

The current seizure classification [45] (Table 3.1) is more clearly related to seizure experience and the parts of the brain involved than older classifications. Seizures are described as either 'partial' or 'generalized', depending upon whether the seizure starts in a localized part of the brain and produces symptoms relating to that part's function, or whether it

Table 3.1 Classification of seizures.

	Old terms
Partial seizures (local onset)	

Simple partial (no impairment of consciousness) May involve. motor symptoms
      sensory/somatosensory symptoms (auras)
      autonomic symptoms
      psychic symptoms
	Jacksonian

Complex partial (impairment of consciousness)	
either simple partial evolving to complex partial	Psychomotor/
or impairment of consciousness from onset	temporal lobe
(abnormal behaviour/sensation:	epilepsy
automatisms, chewing, lip smacking)	
Both simple and complex partial seizures may evolve to become secondarily generalized seizures	
Primary generalized seizures (bilaterally symmetrical, no focal onset)	
Tonic–clonic	Grand mal
Tonic	
Clonic	
Absence	Petit mal
Myoclonic	Absence
Infantile spasms	
Atonic	Drop

Important note: Petit mal absences must be distinguished from attacks involving loss of awareness during complex partial seizures because treatment is different. Petit mal absence has no aura; the onset is abrupt; the absence is very brief and recovery of consciousness is immediate.

involves most of both halves of the brain simultaneously. The diagrams which follow are simple, and may be found useful in explaining the nature of their epilepsy to patients.

Partial seizures (localization-related)

'Partial seizures' may remain localized or spread to involve other parts of the brain and may then evolve to produce a 'secondarily generalized tonic–clonic seizure' (Fig. 3.1). The initial symptoms experienced will depend upon the site of onset and subsequent symptoms will be related to the spread of seizure activity (Fig. 3.2).

Simple partial seizures

'Partial seizures' are described as 'simple partial seizures' if consciousness is unimpaired. There may be motor symptoms if the frontal lobe is involved, physical sensory symptoms from the parietal lobe, visual symptoms from the occipital lobe, and a variety of autonomic and psychic symptoms from the temporal lobe. The 'aura' typically associated with seizures originating in the temporal lobe is regarded as a simple 'somatosensory' partial seizure when it occurs by itself, without spreading to become a complex partial, or a secondarily generalized seizure.

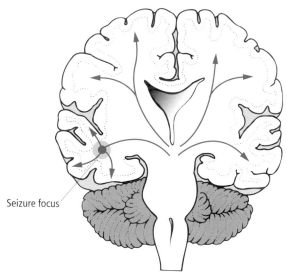

Seizure focus

Fig. 3.1 Diagrammatic representation of the spread of neural activity during a partial seizure developing into a secondarily generalized seizure.

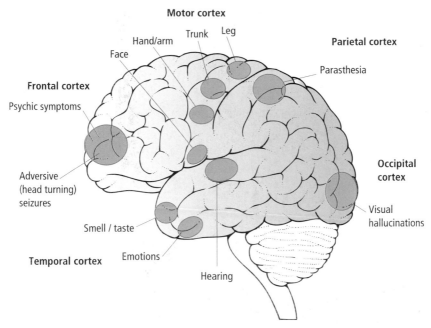

Motor cortex

Hand/arm Trunk Leg

Face

Parietal cortex

Parasthesia

Frontal cortex

Psychic symptoms

Occipital cortex

Adversive (head turning) seizures

Visual hallucinations

Smell / taste

Temporal cortex Emotions

Hearing

Fig. 3.2 The site of seizure onset affects the initial symptoms.

Complex partial seizures

Complex partial seizures are the commonest type of partial seizure, and were previously described as temporal lobe seizures or psychomotor seizures. They can, in fact, arise in the temporal, frontal, parietal and occipital lobes, but rarely originate in the last two.

The presence of some degree of disturbance of consciousness distinguishes complex partial seizures from simple partial seizures. Commonly, the individual will experience a simple partial seizure, such as an olfactory aura or déjà vu, and then appear to be inattentive or staring. This type of loss of awareness is normally more prolonged than the absence of 'petit mal' for which it is often mistaken (many minutes rather than 10–30 seconds). Sometimes this loss of awareness is associated with complex movements such as chewing and may involve semi-purposeful movements such as plucking with fingers or adjusting clothing. In some patients confused or odd behaviour is prolonged, and an individual may appear to be 'loitering with intent', or fail to pay for an item while in a shop (Fig. 3.3).

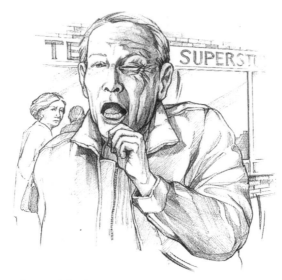

Fig. 3.3 A complex partial seizure.

Partial seizures becoming secondarily generalized seizures

Both simple and complex partial seizures may evolve to become secondarily generalized seizures. For example, the well-known, though rare, 'Jacksonian seizure', the onset of involuntary motor movement without loss of consciousness, is classified as a 'simple motor seizure'. If the seizure then progresses to loss of consciousness with 'tonic–clonic' movements it is described as a 'simple motor seizure with secondary generalization'. The sequence of events illustrates how seizure activity can spread: jerking starts in one thumb, spreads to affect the whole hand, then the arm, the side of the face and finally the leg. Eventually, when the whole of one side of the body is jerking, a tonic–clonic seizure may occur.

An individual may experience different seizure activity at different times, for example an 'olfactory aura' may not always be followed by a 'tonic–clonic' seizure, and one individual may at times experience 'complex partial' seizures which do not go on to secondarily generalize but will do so on other occasions.

Generalized seizures

In generalized seizures, the whole of both hemispheres *appear* to be affected simultaneously. It is probable that seizure activity actually begins in the deeper structures of the brain. This is shown schematically in Fig. 3.4.

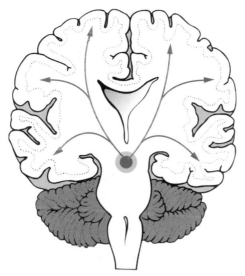

Fig. 3.4 Pattern of neural activity during primary generalized seizures.

Tonic–clonic seizures

Where a 'tonic–clonic' seizure occurs without evidence of focal onset, such as a preceding aura or complex partial seizure, it is regarded as primary generalized from the onset.

Since misdiagnosis of epilepsy is commonly based upon mistakenly assuming abnormal movements associated with loss of consciousness to be tonic–clonic, it is worth describing this type of attack in detail and viewing a video if possible.

The sequence of events is as follows. The **tonic phase** usually lasts 10–20 seconds. There is generalized muscle contraction, beginning with **brief flexion**; the eyes look up, the arms are raised, abducted and externally rotated, with semi-flexion at the elbows (Fig. 3.5). (If the bladder is full, there may be urination.) This is followed by **extension**, which first involves the back and the neck, a tonic cry may occur, the arms extend, the legs extend and become adducted and externally rotated. Breathing stops and there may be cyanosis; **tremor** then begins as relaxation occurs, at first at eight per second coarsening to four per second, leading into the clonic phase.

The **clonic phase** usually lasts about 30 seconds as muscular relaxation completely interrupts the tonic contraction; brief **violent flexor spasms** affect the whole body and the tongue is often bitten.

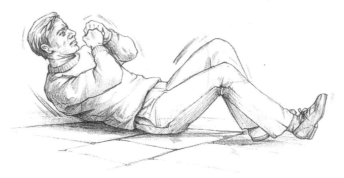

Fig. 3.5 A tonic–clonic seizure.

Simple absence (petit mal)

A common error is to label any attacks exhibiting lack of awareness, such as those associated with complex partial seizures, as petit mal absence. The distinction matters because the treatment is different.

    Petit mal absence is uncommon and tends to affect children, not adults. There is no aura; it has an abrupt onset, is very brief, usually under 10 seconds and rarely more than 30 seconds; the eyelids may flutter and recovery of consciousness is immediate (Fig. 3.6). Brief automatisms, such as lip smacking, can sometimes occur in prolonged attacks, but these are not usually as pronounced as in complex partial seizures.

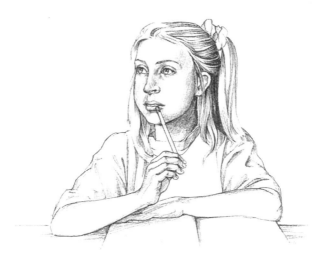

Fig. 3.6 A petit mal absence seizure.

Less-common generalized seizures

1 Atonic attacks (very rare) in which the patient loses muscle tone and falls.

2 Myoclonic seizures characterized by multiple uncontrollable jerks. Patients with these often also have tonic–clonic seizures.

3 Tonic seizures (rare) in which the patient's muscles go stiff and lead to a fall.

Epilepsy syndromes

Classifying epilepsy further into syndromes [46], when it is possible, provides better guidance about prognosis and the choice of treatment than seizure type alone. **An epilepsy syndrome is characterized by a cluster of signs, symptoms and other factors such as an EEG, and especially the age of onset. Most epilepsy syndromes are age-related, occur in childhood** and are best understood by, and the rarer ones managed totally by, specialists. It can nevertheless be helpful for GPs to have a broad understanding and to be able to recognize the commoner syndromes. An initial assessment even by a hospital specialist may be wrong, not least because the full picture may not emerge for some time (see Case study 2 below).

Epilepsy syndromes are classified in four groups (Table 3.2 shows a simplified version). For practical purposes there are two main groups, which follow the same logic as the seizure classification, i.e. idiopathic generalized epilepsies and localization-related epilepsies.

Idiopathic generalized epilepsies

These are mainly genetic in origin, and include childhood absence epilepsy (petit mal), juvenile myoclonic epilepsy and tonic–clonic seizures. Two syndromes are important to recognize: childhood absence epilepsy and juvenile myoclonic epilepsy.

Childhood absence epilepsy

Childhood absence epilepsy covers about 8% of epilepsy in children (absence attacks, petit mal, described above). Only 6% persist into adult life, but tonic–clonic seizures commonly develop in 40–60%, within 5–10 years. **Treatment is specific**, traditionally, with sodium valproate or ethosuximide. Neither carbamazepine nor phenytoin are any use.

Table 3.2 Epilepsy syndromes. A simplified classification.

Localization-related (partial) epilepsies and syndromes
Idiopathic
Benign focal motor epilepsy of childhood
Benign occipital epilepsy of childhood
Symptomatic
Simple partial epilepsies
Complex partial epilepsies
Cryptogenic (presumed symptomatic but aetiology unknown)
Generalized epilepsies
Idiopathic
Childhood absence
Benign myoclonic epilepsy
Tonic–clonic awakening epilepsy
Juvenile myoclonic epilepsy
Symptomatic
Infantile spasms (West's syndrome)
Lennox–Gastaut syndrome
Early myoclonic epilepsies
Unclassified epilepsies and syndromes
Neonatal seizures
Undetermined epilepsies
Specific epileptic syndromes
Situation-related seizures
Febrile convulsions
Acute symptomatic seizures, e.g. metabolic, drugs, alcohol
Reflex epilepsy

Juvenile myoclonic epilepsy

This covers about 6% of all epilepsy; 80% commence between the ages of 12 and 18 years. Myoclonic jerks are usually symmetrical and mainly affect the upper limbs (Fig. 3.7). Absence attacks may also occur. Seizures commonly occur after wakening and are made worse by sleep deprivation; 90% have tonic–clonic seizures and 25% typical absence seizures. Valproate is the drug of choice. **Other drugs may make the condition worse**. Treatment may have to be continued indefinitely, as 90% of patients will relapse if medication is withdrawn. Often this syndrome presents with tonic–clonic seizures and the presence of morning myoclonic attacks may go unrecognized.

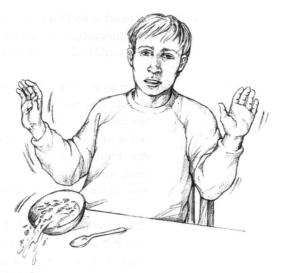

Fig. 3.7 Myoclonic jerks.

Localization-related epilepsies

These have a focus of activity such as scar tissue, giving rise to partial seizures which may spread.

Most epilepsy in adults is focal in origin. Symptomatic or cryptogenic partial epilepsies are the commonest group and include temporal, frontal, parietal and occipital lobe epilepsies. As the terms imply, the aetiologies are known or suspected.

As a result of improvements in imaging, structural lesions are now being identified more often than in the past. Seizures thought to be generalized on clinical grounds may be shown to have a structural cause, and as a consequence there are increasing opportunities for surgical management.

Illustrative case studies

Case study 1

Just over 20 years ago, Margaret, then aged 14 years, was sitting watching television after returning home from school. Suddenly, she was seen to stiffen, she lost consciousness, became blue, her breathing became noisy and she developed violent jerking movements which lasted for a few minutes. She then became limp, pale and sweaty and was unrousable for about 10 minutes. On regaining consciousness she was confused, had no recollection of what had happened; she then fell asleep, and when she awoke she complained of headache, soreness of the jaw and the insides of her cheeks, and had petechial haemorrhages around her eyes.

Margaret was seen within a few weeks by a neurologist. Neurological examination and EEG were normal. The neurologist told her that she had had a 'grand mal' seizure and had 'idiopathic epilepsy'. He added that she would have this for life, she would always need to take tablets, she should not swim, climb, or ride a bike, and would never be able to drive a car. He took well-intentioned pains to ensure that Margaret had a realistic view of the future based on views on prognosis held at the time.

Fortunately, as time went on, Margaret had relatively few seizures, but noticed that they were always preceded by an odd sensation of 'slowing down and going backwards'. In time, her seizures were fully controlled on carbamazepine, and she now leads a full life, including driving a car. She has been free of seizures for 16 years.

Comment

The original seizure description, including events before and after, was typical of a classic 'grand mal' seizure (old terminology), or what is nowadays described as a 'tonic–clonic seizure'. There were no features on this occasion to indicate whether the seizure was 'generalized' from the outset, or was a 'partial seizure' which had evolved from a 'localized' part of the brain. No underlying cause was apparent from the neurological examination or investigations. The nature of her seizures became clearer with time, and the later recognition of an aura preceding the 'tonic–clonic' seizure indicated that the seizures had their source in a localized area of the brain. In other words, a 'simple partial seizure' evolved to become a 'secondarily generalized seizure'. This suggests a temporal lobe epilepsy. Treatment with carbamazepine was appropriate and since Margaret has been seizure-free for a long period, she might consider withdrawing her medication. (But since she has a driver's licence she probably will not.)

Case study 2

Eileen, aged 42 years, started with epilepsy at the age of 13 years. Her seizures at first were tonic–clonic, and typically occurred when first rising in the morning. Occasionally, she had them at night. She had them more often if she was short of sleep. She also had what she called 'minor attacks'. In these, she was briefly unaware and sometimes stuttered. Over the years she was treated with a range of drugs and complained of being tired all the time and having a poor memory. At the age of 32 years, she moved and changed her doctor who reviewed her epilepsy and her treatment. Her tonic–clonic fits then occurred about once a month, her 'stuttering attacks' several times a week. It was concluded that she had partial epilepsy, and that her 'stuttering attacks' were complex partial seizures. Since phenytoin was the only drug that she was taking in a near therapeutic dose, it was agreed that after increasing the latter, other drugs would be withdrawn.

Very quickly, Eileen's general well-being improved. Her tonic–clonic seizures became less frequent, but her 'stuttering attacks', which occurred mainly in the mornings, were only slightly improved. She continued on monotherapy on a maximum dosage of phenytoin for several years, but then developed peripheral neuropathy and her treatment was changed to carbamazepine. Eileen's 'stuttering attacks' then became much worse; if in the kitchen or at table, crockery she was handling would go flying (Fig. 3.8). It became apparent that she was experiencing myoclonic seizures, not complex partial seizures. Eileen really had juvenile myoclonic epilepsy and her treatment was changed to sodium valproate with good results.

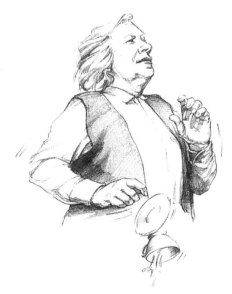

Fig. 3.8 Myoclonic seizures.

Comment

This case shows how the true nature of juvenile myoclonic epilepsy can be missed and how rewarding it is to keep it in mind and treat it effectively. It supports the arguments for syndromic classification.

Making the Diagnosis: Is it Epilepsy? 4

Chapter 3 pointed to the need to consider the diagnosis of epilepsy at three levels: the underlying cause, seizure type and epilepsy syndrome. It also emphasized the primary importance of the clinical history. In practice, many clinicians, and certainly most GPs, find making a diagnosis of epilepsy difficult. The major difficulty lies in distinguishing epilepsy from other paroxysmal disorders which result in convulsions, or loss of consciousness or awareness.

As many as 26% of patients referred to specialist epilepsy centres with a diagnosis of epilepsy do not have epilepsy [22]. Scheepers *et al.*, in a specialist review of 214 patients with a diagnosis of epilepsy in general practice, found a misdiagnosis rate of 23.8% [23]. Of the 49 misdiagnosed, 7 had suffered a single seizure only, 15 a cardiovascular cause, 5 a cerebro-vascular cause, 6 were alcohol related, 3 migraine, 2 post-anaesthetic, 1 pre-eclamptic, and 10 had psychogenic non-epileptic seizures (see 'Pseudo-seizures and non-epileptic attack disorder', page 38).

Patients misdiagnosed as having epilepsy have often been treated as having epilepsy for years, by GPs, general physicians, paediatricians and junior staff. Commonly, the mistake was made at the outset, with an inadequate history and later the application of the label 'known epileptic'.

So, if hospital doctors often get the diagnosis wrong, it must be very, very difficult? Well, yes and no. Mostly it should be easy, and very occasionally it is not. The key to getting it right is a full history, including recent witnessed accounts of possible seizures and of events surrounding them. There are specific features in clinical presentations which should strongly suggest syncope (Table 4.1) and migraine rather than epilepsy. The GP, or other clinician first involved, has the best chance of getting this crucial information. Tests have their place in identifying non-epilepsy causes, and in the classification of epilepsy and in detecting underlying causes, but the diagnosis is first and foremost a clinical one. After that, co-operation between different specialists—neurologists, cardiologists and psychiatrists—may be needed to ensure accuracy of diagnosis.

This chapter outlines the initial work-up and actions, considers the differential diagnosis of epilepsy, and outlines principles to help get the diagnosis right.

Initial work-up

The following should be sought:
1 A description of any attacks thought to be epileptic—**witnessed accounts are crucial**;
2 Other neurological symptoms;
3 Presence of seizures in infancy or childhood;
4 Family history of epilepsy or febrile convulsions;
5 A history of neurological problems, e.g. birth trauma, head injury or meningitis;
6 Physical examination to exclude neurological or other abnormality;
7 A developmental history in children.

Initial action

Referral

New cases suspected of having epilepsy should be seen by a neurologist or physician/paediatrician with expertise in epilepsy; ideally within 4 weeks, because of the understandable anxiety.

Urgent referral

Severe, prolonged, very frequent seizures, or focal neurological signs, should lead to urgent referral or admission.

Starting treatment

Treatment is not usual after a single seizure, but is advisable if a patient experiences more than one attack in a year. Treatment is best deferred for specialist advice, but if the diagnosis is not in doubt, and treatment has to be started while waiting, consult the section on 'Choosing the right anti-epileptic drug' (Chapter 5).

Initial counselling

A full counselling checklist is shown in Chapter 8, pages 110 and 111.

1 Advice to relatives about what to do during a fit.

2 Advice regarding driving, driving regulations and avoidance of danger.

3 Consider referring to a specialist epilepsy liaison nurse if available and to the British Epilepsy Association or other patient organization (see 'Sources of Help and Advice', Appendix 1).

Principles in diagnosing epilepsy

It is often possible to make a seizure diagnosis, an aetiological diagnosis and classify by syndrome from the medical history alone.

The clinical history should lead to the seizure diagnosis. This depends particularly upon a witnessed description of events, before, during and after a suspected seizure. Recognizing the seizure type will then often indicate the underlying source or aetiology, and taken with other factors such as age or test results provide a syndromic classification.

Case study 3

Jackie, aged 25 years, had a tonic–clonic seizure one morning while getting her children ready for school. Her husband was present and was able to give a very full description of the incident. Jackie, at the time 8 weeks' pregnant, was taken straight to hospital and sent home with a diagnosis of 'idiopathic epilepsy', with instructions that she should start on phenytoin if she should have any further seizures.

On the face of it, this was reasonable. Certainly, one seizure is not enough to justify a diagnosis of epilepsy. However, on checking the story, it emerged that immediately before losing consciousness, Jackie recalled having a feeling of 'déjà vu'. Not only that, she remembered similar, identical sensations of 'déjà vu' on three or four mornings over the previous 6 months, but without loss of consciousness.

Comment

A first tonic–clonic seizure at Jackie's age was most likely to be focal in onset, whereas in a child or teenager, the possibility of a primary generalized epilepsy might be a consideration. In the event, the history of 'déjà vu' pointed clearly to a simple partial seizure with secondary generalization, and therefore probably a temporal lobe focus, and so temporal lobe epilepsy. An EEG later identified a possible focus in the left temporal lobe.

Misdiagnosis is common but can be avoided

Misdiagnoses commonly result from a failure to distinguish epileptic seizures from simple faints or other cardiovascular causes of loss of consciousness, especially in newly presenting cases. The occurrence of urinary incontinence or twitching movements can in particular lead to a mistaken diagnosis of epilepsy. Of patients with apparently intractable epilepsy, a number turn out not to have epilepsy, but to have non-epileptic attacks or pseudo-seizures (termed 'non-epileptic attack disorder', NEAD). Sometimes patients with pseudo-seizures also have a true history of epilepsy.

Case study 4: epilepsy or syncope?

Lynne, 23 years old and 14 weeks' pregnant, came to the surgery with her boyfriend and asked to be seen. She was extremely distressed, complained of feeling ill, off-balance and of having a headache. A few days earlier she had attended a hospital outpatients department, following referral by a partner in the practice because of a series of 'blackouts'. She had attended hospital with her mother because her boyfriend was at work. The medical registrar at the hospital told her that she had 'grand mal epilepsy', and had prescribed phenytoin at a dose of 400 mg daily which she started straight away.

Lynne wanted to know what epilepsy was, she thought that the pills were upsetting her and was frightened about the dangers of the treatment for her unborn baby. Apparently, since becoming pregnant, she had experienced a number of attacks of loss of consciousness, during some of which she had been incontinent of urine. Nowhere in the notes or reports was there a description of an attack.

On enquiring, it became clear that during none of her attacks had she lost consciousness suddenly. In every instance she had been standing, felt 'empty in the head', nauseated and sometimes hot. On several occasions she had time to go from her living room to her kitchen to get a glass of water. Sometimes she felt better as a result and did not pass out. When she did lose consciousness, her boyfriend said that she flopped and went pale. There was no stiffness and no jerking. Twitching and incontinence had occurred when the boyfriend had held her upright during the attacks.

The couple were told that the attacks were not due to epilepsy, but to fainting attacks associated with pregnancy. Lynne could stop the medication. She was advised to avoid prolonged standing and to put her feet up if she felt faint again. She had no further attacks.

Comment

Most misdiagnoses, like this one, result from a failure to distinguish epilepsy from faints or other cardiovascular causes of loss of consciousness. Epilepsy is usually characterized by abruptness of onset, whereas syncope, as in Lynne's case, is often preceded by quite prolonged symptoms of light-headedness. In epilepsy, attacks are usually brief and tend to be stereotyped. Lynne had time to move about the house and her attacks varied—she did not always pass out. True, she wet herself and twitched a bit, but twitching and incontinence of micturition can occur in syncope, especially if the victim is held upright. In tonic–clonic seizures (see Chapter 3, page 25), the commonest type of seizure to be confused with syncope, movements are very marked, even violent, and recovery can be slow, with confusion, headache and sleepiness. Lynne recovered quickly. Table 4.1 shows the main differences between syncope and epilepsy.

Case study 5: all not what it seemed

Linda had been diagnosed with epilepsy at the age of 15 years. There were well-described tonic–clonic seizures preceded by an unpleasant

Table 4.1 The differences between syncope and epileptic seizures. Modified from Laidlaw, J., Richens, A. and Chadwick, D. (eds) *A Textbook of Epilepsy*, 4th edn. Edinburgh: Churchill Livingstone, 1993.

	Syncope	Seizures
Posture	Upright	Any posture
Pallor and sweating	Invariably present	Uncommon
Onset	Gradual	Sudden/aura
Injury	Rare	Not uncommon
Convulsive jerks	Not uncommon	Common
Incontinence	Sometimes	Common
Unconsciousness	Seconds	Minutes
Recovery	Rapid	Often slow
Post-ictal confusion	Rare	Common
Frequency	Infrequent	May be frequent
Precipitating factors	Crowded places	Rare
	Lack of food	
	Unpleasant circumstances	
	Pain	

Note: These differences are not always helpful in distinguishing syncope from epileptic seizures in childhood or the elderly.

frightened feeling. Her EEG had a temporal lobe focus, and she had skin lesions of tuberous sclerosis suggesting the aetiology. The diagnosis was not much in doubt and her seizures were partly controlled on medication.

A timid, dependent woman, she had married a rather domineering husband who worked away, and they had a child. Linda continued to report occasional seizures despite what appeared to be optimum treatment with different anti-epileptics; occasionally she would end up in the accident and emergency department, but never seemed to hurt herself. She developed a disabling, chronic back problem and a limp, which were thought by orthopaedic consultants to be hysterical.

The strong suspicion that the attacks were not epileptic was confirmed on an urgently requested home visit for repeated seizures. Linda was in bed looking fine, her husband was home for the weekend looking fed up. After taking a history of events, the couple were told that the attacks did not sound like epilepsy. Linda promptly had an attack. She looked upwards and away, started jerking her body and then her limbs, and rolling around the bed. Her movements were uneven and flailing and persisted for several minutes, they eased off briefly when the view was expressed that this was certainly not epilepsy and then resumed with greater vigour for a few more minutes. Linda recovered quite quickly from her 'attack', and once the true nature of her 'seizures' was recognized her 'seizure control' improved.

Comment

Linda's attack during the home visit was provoked by suggestion, she averted her gaze, her movements were unlike those of a tonic–clonic seizure, they were prolonged and altered in response to hearing the doctor's comments. Her previous attacks were unassociated with injury. Identifying 'non-epileptic seizures' and dealing with the problem once it is recognized can be far from easy, even less so when the patient has epilepsy. Table 4.2 shows the main differences between epileptic seizures and pseudo-seizures, now more commonly referred to as 'non-epileptic attack disorder' (NEAD).

Pseudo-seizures and non-epileptic attack disorder

The term 'non-epileptic attack disorder' (NEAD) has come to replace the better known labels psychogenic seizures or pseudo-seizures to describe, as Betts and Boden [47] put it, 'the occurrence of paroxysmal attacks which resemble epileptic and other organic attacks, but are devoid of clinical or EEG features associated with epilepsy and/or other organic cause'.

Clinicians and nurses who diagnose non-epileptic seizures often feel angry that they have been deceived by a patient manufacturing symptoms. In fact, **the vast majority of psychogenic non-epileptic seizures are beyond the control of the patient**. They often arise from subconscious events, cause severe social disruption, and can cause significant injuries. Once diagnosed correctly the majority can eventually, with psychiatric treatment, become free from attacks and also unnecessary anti-epileptic medication.

People diagnosed with NEAD have generally personally experienced a seizure or seizures in infancy (febrile or epileptic), or observed a family member or close friend who experienced seizures. Many of those referred

Table 4.2 The differences between epileptic seizures and pseudo-seizures. From Laidlaw, J., Richens, A. and Chadwick, D. (eds) *A Textbook of Epilepsy*, 4th edn. Edinburgh: Churchill Livingstone, 1993.

	Epileptic seizure	Pseudo-seizures
Onset	Sudden	May be gradual
Retained consciousness in prolonged seizure	Very rare	Common
Pelvic thrusting	Rare	Common
Flailing, thrashing, asynchronous limb movements	Rare	Common
Rolling movements	Rare	Common
Cyanosis	Common	Unusual
Tongue-biting and other injury	Common	Less common
Stereotyped attacks	Usual	Uncommon
Duration	Seconds or minutes	Often many minutes
Gaze aversion	Rare	Common
Resistance to passive limb movement or eye-opening	Unusual	Common
Prevention of hand falling on to face	Unusual	Common
Induced by suggestion	Rarely	Often
Post-ictal drowsiness or confusion	Usual	Often absent
Ictal EEG abnormality	Almost always	Never
Post-ictal EEG abnormal (after seizure with impairment of consciousness)	Usually	Rarely

to specialist centres with apparently intractable epilepsy have NEAD and most are women, many being frequent attenders of A&E departments. The diagnosis of NEAD is made as a result of the exclusion of epilepsy and other physiological disorders. Attacks are often bizarre in comparison to epileptic seizures, making it relatively easy for an expert to distinguish between them —but difficult for the rest of us. (A handy camcorder can make up for the lack of immediacy of the expert.) Table 4.2 shows the main differences.

The problem for the generalist in finding or suspecting the diagnosis of NEAD in an individual is finding the appropriate specialist to help.

Occasionally the diagnosis is missed

The diagnosis may be missed if the patient experiences only absence attacks or complex partial seizures. Childhood absence epilepsy may not be recognized in children who do not also develop tonic–clonic seizures and attacks may have a marked effect on school performance. Obviously, the GP is reliant on parents or teachers realizing that something is amiss. Complex partial seizures occur in both children and adults, and can in the former be confused with absence attacks; they are, however, usually more prolonged and automatisms last longer and should be easier to spot.

Case study 6: one that nearly got away

Fred, 68 years old, a frequent surgery attender with arthritis, started to complain of dizzy attacks. He was cheerful, slightly deaf and forgetful, and always accompanied by his attentive but rather vague wife. His neck was very stiff, and he said he got dizzy when he looked up. His wife was only able to say 'well, he just gets dizzy'. It was concluded that Fred had problems with his vertebrobasilar circulation, and it was rather left at that.

One day, a home visit was requested for another member of the family. During the visit, Fred was noticed to turn his head to one side and begin making chewing movements. He was quite unresponsive for several minutes, and on recovery had no idea what had been happening. His wife said, 'Well, he's always like that when he's dizzy. It happens a lot.'

Fred's complex partial seizures were greatly reduced, though not completely controlled, by treatment with carbamazepine.

Comment

This illustrates the difficulty of recognizing partial seizures in patients who never have secondarily generalized tonic–clonic seizures. Partial seizures tend to be harder to bring under control than tonic–clonic seizures, and some patients prefer to put up with them rather than take pills.

If seizures are classified wrongly the treatment might end up being wrong

Although most major anti-epileptic drugs are effective against most types of seizure, and particularly against tonic–clonic seizures, some of the epilepsy syndromes starting in childhood respond differently. Childhood absence (petit mal) and the myoclonus of juvenile myoclonic epilepsy, for example, do not respond to either phenytoin or carbamazepine. In fact, carbamazepine may make myoclonus worse. Sodium valproate is effective in these conditions, and ethosuximide specifically in absence.

Case study 2

Eileen, who featured in Chapter 3 (page 30), developed epilepsy at the age of 13 years. Her attacks included tonic–clonic attacks which occurred typically in the morning, or when she was short of sleep. She also had attacks in which she was briefly unaware and stuttered. These were initially and at later review thought to be complex partial seizures. Anti-epileptic drugs controlled her tonic–clonic seizures fairly well, but her other attacks continued to be a problem. A change of medication to carbamazepine after many years led to a worsening of her so-called 'stuttering attacks', which were only then recognized as myoclonic jerks. It became clear that she had unrecognized juvenile myoclonic epilepsy. This eventually responded to sodium valproate.

Comment

Juvenile myoclonic epilepsy comprises about 6% of epilepsy, perhaps two in an average group practice. It may be worthwhile checking to see.

Time often makes the diagnosis clearer

It is easy to criticize those who do not quite get the seizure diagnosis right when a patient first presents. One wonders how epilepsy specialists would get on if they actually saw patients within a short time of the onset of seizures. The passage of time was featured in clarifying the seizure diagnoses in all of the cases described here, except Lynne (Case study 4) who did not have epilepsy. Time spent with Lynne did, however, prevent a mistake.

It is important to review the diagnosis in patients whose seizures are poorly controlled

Although compliance is the most likely reason for poor seizure control, it may be that the patient does not have epilepsy, or the attacks are not all epileptic, as in the case of Linda (Case study 5). It may be that an underlying neurological cause deserves attention.

A mistaken diagnosis of epilepsy may mean that something else is missed

It is bad enough to be labelled as having epilepsy, but a treatable life-threatening cause of recurring unconsciousness such as cardiac syncope in the elderly may be overlooked. (Syncope due to ventricular tachycardia untreated has a mortality of 30%.)

The role of the EEG, computed tomography (CT) and magnetic resonance imaging (MRI)

(See Chapter 9, page 126, for patient information.)

So far, a great deal has been said about clinical diagnosis, witnessed accounts of what might be seizures, and little about investigations. Investigations are important, may be supportive of the diagnosis and may identify underlying pathology, but are secondary to the clinical diagnosis.

The role of the EEG

The routine inter-ictal EEG is often misinterpreted, particularly in children. Minor abnormalities may be used to support an unsatisfactory diagnosis of epilepsy when there is clinical uncertainty. As many as 10–15% of the normal population have non-specific EEG abnormalities, and patients with undoubted seizures may have normal inter-ictal EEGs [48].

The EEG can contribute to the classification of an individual's epilepsy, help to clarify his or her prognosis and indicate the choice of treatment; for example, in absence attacks where the presence of generalized spike wave abnormalities helps to distinguish childhood absence from complex partial seizures, or in sleep or awakening tonic–clonic seizures, where the EEG can often demonstrate whether seizures are likely to be primary or secondarily generalized. Focal changes on the EEG may also arouse suspicion of a structural lesion.

Ambulatory EEGs, combined with audio-visual telemetry, are important in evaluating patients with severe epilepsy and in excluding pseudo-seizures (NEAD).

Special EEGs, with depth electrodes, are used in investigating patients being considered for surgery, in order to define epileptogenic foci.

CT and MRI

Neither CT nor MRI scanning are routine for all cases of epilepsy. They are particularly indicated where there is evidence of focal onset, e.g. adults presenting with partial seizures with or without neurological signs and/or focal abnormality on an EEG. Other indications are epilepsy unresponsive to anti-epileptics, epilepsy which is worsening and new or progressive neurological signs and/or symptoms.

MRI is far more sensitive than CT, it is more expensive, not readily available and is mainly used for patients being considered for surgery.

There is no point in scanning where there was a clear diagnosis of primary generalized epilepsy.

Conclusions: how to get it right

GPs quite properly look to specialists for help in making the diagnosis of epilepsy. However, access to a specialist with particular expertise in epilepsy in the UK is the exception rather than the rule, and other hospital doctors with variable expertise are often involved. The best contribution that the GP can make, whoever he or she has to work with, is to ensure that the story is right, and in particular to obtain witnessed accounts of possible seizures. Occasionally, it may be necessary to challenge the opinions of others (see Case study 4, page 36). Finally, there is immense value in keeping patients under review and being prepared to reconsider the diagnosis, ideally of course with specialist help. It is not actually all that difficult and is quite interesting and rewarding to do.

5 Treatment: General Principles, Anti-Epileptic Drug Therapy, Surgery and Other Treatment

Treatment is more than controlling seizures

Once a diagnosis of epilepsy has been made, the doctor naturally wants to get on with stopping the fits. The seizure type and possibly also a syndrome have been recognized, and any underlying pathological cause requiring treatment in its own right has been considered. The time to prescribe seems to have arrived. But the effective treatment of epilepsy entails far more than choosing an appropriate anti-epileptic drug. Epilepsy, perhaps more than any other chronic illness, carries unique burdens and consequences for patients and relatives. Apart from the experience of the seizures, which is bad enough, there is the effect of having epilepsy, of felt or actual stigma; there may be an associated handicap such as learning disability, and, for many, considerable problems with social life and employment.

So, although for doctors the questions 'What drug do I choose for a newly diagnosed patient?', 'How do I go about changing drugs for a poorly controlled patient?', 'Can drugs be stopped safely?', 'When?', 'How?' tend to be of immediate and primary concern, for patients and families, when epilepsy is newly diagnosed, the questions at the forefront are more likely to be: 'What is epilepsy?', 'Will she die in one of these attacks?', 'Is it a tumour on the brain or a haemorrhage?', 'Will it lead to mental illness?', 'Will I be able to drive?', 'What about my job?' It is as important to identify and respond to these immediate worries as it is to instruct about treatment. For a new patient, immediate issues are likely to include safety and support, for example, what to do in a fit, driving regulations, sport, sources of information and counselling. But only so much can be taken in at one time, and any attempt to give too much information at the same time as the diagnosis is explained is likely to fail.

What is relevant may change. The implications of having epilepsy are different not only for individuals but also for the same individual at different times. For example, the difficulties for a 15-year-old schoolgirl who is a keen swimmer will change a few years later when she wants to hold a driver's licence, certainly when she considers oral contraception and again later if she wants to have children.

We should aim then, not only to prescribe anti-epileptic medication effectively, but as we do so, remember to inform patients and families about epilepsy, its treatment and consequences, so that they can be independent and live life as fully as possible. It is helpful to have a checklist available (see Chapter 8, pages 110 and 111) both for newly diagnosed patients and when reviewing those with established epilepsy.

Drug therapy is the mainstay of treatment. It is usually tried first and is the main purpose of this chapter. Surgery, which is becoming increasingly an option for poorly controlled epilepsy, and alternative treatments such as biofeedback and aromatherapy, are referred to at the end of this chapter.

When should a GP prescribe?

All right, you have contributed to getting the diagnosis right! You can see that it is quite appropriate to give information out, ensure that patients and relatives have explanations and opportunities to ask questions. And much of this can take place when issuing a prescription. But, how much can a GP be expected to take on? Should a GP, in any circumstances, start treatment in a newly diagnosed patient, or for that matter challenge a hospital recommendation? Should he or she review, and alter, an established drug regime in a chronic patient? And if a GP's role is mainly to issue prescriptions on the advice of a specialist, how much knowledge about anti-epilepsy drugs does he or she really need?

These are important questions. Obviously, if there is a comprehensive epilepsy service just up the road, with waiting times of weeks rather than months, it is pointless to start or change treatment without advice. The chances are, however, that you will not be so fortunate, and will have to work with what you have got. And, so **where there are delays in getting an expert opinion in a newly diagnosed patient, where there is no doubt about the diagnosis, seizures continue, and the patient wishes, consideration should be given to starting treatment.** Similarly, **where seizures or side-effects continue to cause problems for chronic epilepsy patients the adequacy or appropriateness of treatment should be questioned.**

Potentially, 70–80% of newly diagnosed patients can have their epilepsy controlled. Most of them are controlled on one drug, and a few will remit. At any one time, almost half of a GP's patients with epilepsy will be well controlled, though perhaps encountering drug side-effects. Of the remainder, most will have infrequent seizures, monthly or less, but enough to disrupt life. The latter can often be helped significantly. About one-fifth to one-third of the total will have frequent seizures and be difficult to control, and may best be helped by an epileptologist.

Starting treatment in a newly diagnosed patient—considerations

A decision to start treatment in an individual should take into account the patient's wishes, the type and severity of the attacks and their number and frequency.

The most common scenario demanding action is that of recurring tonic–clonic seizures. In the UK, neurologists would not advocate treatment after a single tonic–clonic seizure, but would after two or more seizures occurring close together, or within a year. A patient with infrequent tonic–clonic seizures occurring only during sleep might prefer not to take medication, but should be warned of the risk of experiencing daytime attacks. Patients experiencing rare partial seizures without secondary generalization might prefer to put up with them.

Epilepsies in early childhood can cause particular difficulties in diagnosis, and one should hesitate further before considering starting treatment while awaiting a specialist opinion.

Challenging therapy started elsewhere—considerations

Patients starting with epilepsy do not necessarily see their GP first. Commonly, they will end up in an accident and emergency department, perhaps being admitted. Bear in mind that where hospital services for epilepsy are provided by general physicians and paediatricians, they do not necessarily have expertise in epilepsy, and important decisions about diagnosis and treatment may be taken by junior staff. They can, and do, get it wrong, and the initial error can lead to serious consequences, not least being incorrectly labelled with a diagnosis of epilepsy with all of the problems that can bestow. Thus, it is important for a GP to query treatment instituted or recommended elsewhere.

The following are examples in which a GP might intervene.

Case studies 3 and 4

The two patients, Lynne and Jackie described in Chapter 4, were both diagnosed as having epilepsy when seen in hospital. Lynne had complicated syncope mistaken for epilepsy, and Jackie was considered to have had a single tonic–clonic seizure due to idiopathic epilepsy.

Both were recommended phenytoin treatment. Although this was a few years ago, phenytoin was not a good idea even then, particularly as both were pregnant and Lynne turned out not to have epilepsy anyway.

As you will recall, Jackie did have epilepsy. A tonic–clonic seizure had led to her attending casualty. Shortly afterwards, it emerged that immediately before her seizure she had experienced a feeling of déjà vu, and recalled similar experiences on four previous occasions, but without loss of consciousness. The diagnosis of epilepsy was not in doubt, but there was strong evidence that she had partial epilepsy, she was in early pregnancy, and it seemed sensible to start treatment while awaiting a specialist opinion. It was **a question of choosing a drug to suit the seizure type, and choosing to suit the patient**. Carbamazepine was appropriate for the seizure type, and it was preferable for a woman who was pregnant, and who might become pregnant again in the future.

Reviewing treatment in chronic epilepsy—considerations

The notion of reviewing patients with chronic epilepsy in general practice with a view to making changes to treatment is challenging and controversial. There is no doubt that most patients in this category will benefit from a review, whether they are experiencing seizures or not. Many will never have had adequate explanations or advice, and will invariably welcome an opportunity to ask questions. Some will be on polytherapy, suffering drug side-effects. In some, with poor control, it may be apparent that treatment is, in modern terms, inappropriate or inadequate. Few GPs may, however, feel up to embarking on major changes without expert advice, and some patients will prefer to have their tablets left as they are, especially if seizure-free and driving. It is, however, worth recognizing opportunities to reduce side-effects and seizures. Some patients may be amenable to minor changes in current medication by the GP, others worthy of referral. If there is no local service, consideration should be given to referring to a special centre even if it means an extra-contractual referral (ECR).

Why you might need to know more about anti-epileptic drugs

1 To start treatment for a newly diagnosed patient when seizures continue, when there is no doubt about the diagnosis and there are delays in getting an epilepsy specialist opinion.

2 To be able to make do, and react appropriately where there is no specialist epilepsy service handy, and available expertise is uncertain.

3 To recognize side-effects, and interactions between old and new anti-epileptic drugs and other drugs.

4 To recognize opportunities to reduce seizures and side-effects in chronic patients.

5 To collaborate in a treatment plan with specialists.

About anti-epileptic drugs

Fortunately, there is no need to understand exactly how anti-epileptic drugs work in order to use them, although it interesting that drugs developed recently were designed with specific mechanisms of action in mind. Logically, this should lead to our using anti-epileptic drugs selectively in the future.

What matters is what the individual drugs do; how they behave, or for that matter misbehave, and most of all what they achieve.

Drug side-effects

No anti-epileptic medication is without side-effects. Earlier drugs, particularly phenobarbitone and phenytoin, were markedly sedative, and were frequently used in combination, which added to the problem. Many patients remain on these drugs as well as being given newer drugs. Patient surveys [43] show that many patients feel that their medication affects them mentally.

Drug interactions

Apart from side-effects, drug interactions can create problems between anti-epileptics themselves, as well as with other medication taken concurrently. Competition for plasma protein binding causes some difficulties, but most interactions are to do with effects on liver metabolism. Three of the major anti-epileptic drugs—phenobarbitone, phenytoin and carbamazepine—are all potent liver 'enzyme inducers', as is the recent arrival, oxcarbazepine. They increase the metabolism of each other when given in combination and alter the metabolism of other drugs. Carbamazepine even induces its own metabolism.

As a consequence, if during polytherapy involving these drugs one is withdrawn, this can lead to toxic levels of the remaining drug. The most important example of other drugs being affected is that of the combined oral contraceptive pill. Phenytoin, carbamazepine and the newer drugs, oxcarbazepine and topiramate, induce the metabolism of oestrogen and this can lead to pill failure. The solution, dealt with later, is to increase the dose of oestrogen. Lamotrigine, although relatively free from side-effects when given alone, has important interactions with both sodium valproate and carbamazepine.

Whether starting treatment in newly diagnosed patients or reviewing chronic patients, our aim is to find the most effective drug for the type of epilepsy, which is also suitable for the individual patient, and further, to use one drug if possible, and secure optimum seizure control on the smallest dose and with the minimum of side-effects.

Choosing the right anti-epileptic drug

Seizure type and, when identifiable, the epilepsy syndrome, should guide the choice of drug. In certain instances, for example, childhood absence epilepsy (petit mal) and juvenile myoclonic epilepsy, sodium valproate is the only major first-line drug to be effective and the choice is crucial (lamotrigine and the new drug levetiracetam are also proving effective). Ethosuximide is only effective in childhood absence epilepsy. Apart from these examples, there is little to choose between the anti-epileptic drugs in common use in terms of effectiveness in treating the two main groups of seizure disorder, **idiopathic generalized epilepsies** and **localization-related epilepsies** (partial, focal). The final choice depends upon the needs of the patient, ease of use and the likelihood of unwanted side-effects.

Choice of drug, apart from childhood absence epilepsy, juvenile myoclonic epilepsy and rare childhood epilepsy syndromes, is mainly determined by the needs of the patient, ease of use and the likelihood of unwanted side-effects.

First- and second-line drugs

In the past, since all have proved effective in treating tonic–clonic seizures and partial seizures, phenobarbitone, phenytoin, carbamazepine and valproate have all been regarded as first-line drugs. Phenobarbitone has, over the years, fallen into disuse because of its side-effects. Phenytoin continues to be prescribed for new patients, but really should not be, given its side-effects and difficulties in use. Nowadays, since sodium valproate and carbamazepine have established themselves as effective drugs with fewer side-effects, phenobarbitone and phenytoin are no longer regarded as suitable drugs of first choice for newly diagnosed epilepsy, but remain important alternatives in managing chronic epilepsy as second-line drugs. Until recently used as an add-on drug, lamotrigine can now be regarded as a second-line drug together with a newcomer to the UK, oxcarbazepine, which is closely related to carbamazepine and similar in efficacy. So at present:

First-line drugs: sodium valproate, carbamazepine.
Second-line drugs: phenytoin, oxcarbazepine, lamotrigine.

New anti-epileptics—add-on drugs

After many years without new anti-epileptic drugs, there has been a steady stream: vigabatrin (1989), lamotrigine (1991), gabapentin (1993), topiramate (1995), tiagabine (1998), and most recently oxcarbazepine (2000) and levetiracetam (2000). Even though non-specialists are unlikely to initiate their use just yet, it is important to know of their usefulness and problems, and these are reviewed in detail in Chapter 6.

Of these, vigabatrin has proved very effective in infantile spasms, and as an add-on in refractory partial seizures, but has little effect in generalized epilepsy, and has many unfortunate side-effects. Gabapentin has proved useful as add-on therapy in partial or secondarily generalized seizures, but not so much in generalized seizure disorders; it has few side-effects and overall it has modest efficacy. Lamotrigine is effective in both partial and generalized seizures including absence and myoclonus; it is regarded by some specialist as a first-line drug. Topiramate is a powerful new drug with a wide spectrum of anti-epileptic activity, but a high rate of side-effects. Tiagabine has mainly been used as add-on therapy in partial epilepsy and its role is not yet clear. Oxcarbazepine, though new to the UK, has been in use abroad for many years; it is closely related to carbamazepine, is similar in effectiveness, but has fewer side-effects. Levetiracetam is a highly effective new drug with a wide spectrum of activity, including juvenile myoclonic epilepsy, and has a low side-effect profile.

Choosing to suit the seizure

Table 5.1 shows the main anti-epileptic drugs for different seizure types. The division of seizures and epilepsy syndromes into those which have focal onset (localization-related) and those which are primary generalized, has implications for anti-epileptic drug choice. When patients present with epilepsy, most commonly with tonic–clonic seizures, the underlying nature of the epilepsy, that is whether it is primary generalized or focal in onset, may not yet be clear.

Table 5.1 Choosing to suit the seizure.

Seizure type	First-line drugs	Second-line drugs	Add-on drugs
Partial seizures			
Simple	Carbamazepine	Phenytoin*	Clobazam
Complex partial			Topiramate
Secondary generalized	Sodium valproate	Phenobarbitone†	Clonazepam
		Lamotrigine	
		Oxcarbazepine	Vigabatrin
	Lamotrigine		Gabapentin
			Levetiracetam
Generalized seizures			
Tonic–clonic	Carbamazepine	Phenytoin*	Clobazam
(grand mal)	Sodium valproate	Phenobarbitone†	Clonazepam
	Lamotrigine	Oxcarbazepine	
Absence	Sodium valproate		
(petit mal)	Ethosuximide		
	Lamotrigine		
Myoclonic,	Sodium valproate		Piracetam
including juvenile	Clonazepam		
myoclonic epilepsy	Lamotrigine		

* Should be avoided in childhood.
† As a last resort.

Partial seizures (and localization-related epilepsies)

All first- and second-line drugs are effective. Carbamazepine and sodium valproate have been found to be equally effective, but there is a general acceptance that carbamazepine is more effective in complex partial seizures. Since these are harder to control than secondarily generalized tonic–clonic seizures, some experts prefer to use carbamazepine where epilepsy is thought to be of focal onset, and especially when partial seizures are a feature.

Primary generalized seizures (idiopathic generalized epilepsies)

Sodium valproate is usually recommended as the treatment of choice in this group because, although carbamazepine and phenytoin are effective against tonic–clonic seizures, they are ineffective in absence and myoclonic epilepsies. **It is important to recognize juvenile myoclonic epilepsy** (see above) **in this respect**, since carbamazepine can make myoclonic attacks worse. Otherwise, carbamazepine and valproate are equally effective for idiopathic generalized tonic–clonic seizures or partial seizures. Ethosuximide is a useful alternative to sodium valproate in children with absence seizures only. Lamotrigine has been found to be effective in absence and myoclonic seizures and should be considered when sodium valproate is not effective, or not tolerated. The new drug levetiracetam is effective in photosensitive epilepsy, myoclonic jerks, and juvenile myoclonic epilepsy refractory to valproate or lamotrigine. Piracetam is effective in myoclonus only.

Choosing to suit the patient

Sedative side-effects are undesirable for anyone, but especially for children in education. For this reason, phenobarbitone and phenytoin are rarely used. The problems of use and the cosmetic side-effects of phenytoin are also a major disadvantage.

The main choice these days, for newly diagnosed epilepsy, lies between carbamazepine and sodium valproate, and the main issues are associated with the differing effects of these two drugs when taken by girls and women. As far as males are concerned, since sodium valproate has the broadest spectrum of action and no particular disadvantages, it is a rational first choice.

For women, choice will be influenced by the need for contraceptive drugs, the possibility of pregnancy, and the effects of valproate on sex hormone levels resulting in anovulatory cycles, amenorrhoea and polycystic ovary syndrome. Additionally, some young women experience marked weight gain on sodium valproate.

The particular problems for women with epilepsy are dealt with more fully in Chapter 7, but the following should be considered when deciding to start or change treatment.

Contraception

Contraception is dealt with in detail in Chapter 7, pages 95–96. The main potential problem is with those drugs (carbamazepine, oxcarbazepine, topiramate, phenytoin and barbiturates) which induce liver enzymes, and therefore increase the metabolism of oestrogens and progestogens, rendering the combined pill or progestogen-only pill unreliable. **In these circumstances a higher dose of combined pill should be used, or double the dose of the progestogen-only pill. Depot progestogens may be a better choice, given every 10 weeks rather than 12-weekly.**

Pregnancy

Pregnancy and epilepsy are covered fully in Chapter 7, page 96. The main points about medication are as follows. All of the older first- and second-line drugs are known to increase the risk of foetal abnormalities, and the risks from the newer drugs are simply not yet known. Both sodium valproate and carbamazepine have a small increased risk for spina bifida. The risk is reduced if only one drug is being taken, in the smallest effective dose. **Advice should be sought before pregnancy**.

Starting treatment in a newly diagnosed patient

Details about individual drugs are given in Chapter 6. Table 5.2 summarizes the dosage regimes in adults. Table 7.2 (page 90) summarizes the regimes for children.

Before prescribing, the considerations mentioned earlier (Chapter 5, page 45) should apply. **Where there are delays in getting an expert opinion in a newly diagnosed patient, where there is no doubt about the diagnosis, when seizures continue and when the patient wishes it, consideration should be given to starting treatment.**

Whether starting treatment from scratch or changing drugs, the following principles apply.

• **The selected drug should be introduced gradually** in order to limit side-effects. This is particularly important in the case of carbamazepine. There is evidence that patients given lamotrigine are less likely to develop a rash if this drug is introduced very slowly.

• **The aim is to gain control on the smallest dose**. If control is immediate, a maintenance dose at the lower level indicated in Tables 5.2 or 7.2 (page 90) is appropriate.

• **If control is not achieved** on the maximum tolerated dosage, or if there are side-effects, **another first-line drug should be substituted**.

• **No drug should be reduced or stopped until the substituted drug has reached therapeutic levels. Stopping a drug suddenly can provoke withdrawal seizures.** It may be necessary to reduce drugs over weeks or months. (Replacing carbamazepine with oxcarbazepine is an exception and can be done abruptly; see Chapter 6, page 72.)

• **Routine measurement of serum levels is rarely necessary**. It is best to titrate the dose of the drug against clinical response and side-effects. Measurement is helpful to check compliance in those with continuing seizures. The complicated pharmacokinetics of phenytoin may require

Table 5.2 Anti-epileptic drug regimens in adults.

Drug	Starting dose	Maintenance dose	Serum levels
Carbamazepine	100–200 mg o.n. first week, max 2400 mg/day 100–200 mg steps at 1–2 weekly intervals	600–1600 mg/day (taken b.d. or t.d.s.)	15–50 µmol/L
Phenytoin	200 mg o.n., 50–100 mg steps, 2–4 weekly intervals (taken daily)	200–400 mg/day, 25 mg steps monthly (when up to 300 mg daily)	40–80 µmol/L
Sodium valproate	600 mg/day, 200 mg steps every three days	600–1500 mg/day (b.d. or t.d.s.) max. 2500 mg/day	Not helpful 250–700 µmol/L (at 2 h after dose)
Ethosuximide	250 mg/day, 250–500 mg steps every 14 days	750–2000 mg/day	200–600 µmol/L
Vigabatrin	500–1000 mg daily, 250–500 mg steps every 1–2 weeks	1000–2000 mg/day, max. 4000 mg	Not helpful
Lamotrigine			Not helpful
As monotherapy	25 mg/day for 2 weeks, 50 mg/day for 2 weeks	100–200 mg/day	
If on valproate	25 mg on alternate days for 2 weeks, 25 mg/day for 2 weeks, 25 mg steps monthly	100–200 mg/day	
If on other anti-epileptic drugs	50 mg/day for 2 weeks, 50 mg twice daily for 2 weeks, 100 mg steps monthly	200–400 mg/day	
Gabapentin	300 mg first day 300 mg b.d. second day 300 mg t.d.s. third day, then 1200 mg daily in 3 doses	1200–3600 mg/day, max 4800 mg/day	Not helpful
Oxcarbazepine	600 mg/day 600 mg/day steps, weekly intervals	900–2400 mg/day (b.d.)	Not established 50–125 µmol/L
Topiramate	25 mg/day 25 mg/day fortnightly steps to 100 mg/day, then 100 mg fortnightly steps	200–600 mg/day* (b.d.)	Not helpful 6–74 µmol/L
Levetiracetam	500 mg b.d. 500–1000 mg weekly steps	1000–3000 mg/day max 4000 mg/day (b.d.)	Not established

*Higher doses when combined with enzyme-inducing drugs

monitoring of levels when problems occur, especially when attempting to improve control with high dosage.

• **Prescribing by brand name is preferable to generic prescribing.** Best get this sorted out at the start. Although it probably may not matter at all for patients who have been easily controlled on a small dose of a single drug for many years, it is impossible to know who these are at the outset. For many patients, control will depend upon carefully adjusted dosage. Preparations vary in bioavailability, and therefore **it is essential that a patient continues on the same preparation, which can only be ensured by prescribing by brand name**. For an individual to lose his or her driver's licence and all that entails because of a single seizure resulting from a change in a preparation is an appalling prospect. It might lead to litigation and is poor economics.

• **Every patient should have a care plan.** This should, as a minimum, include the proposed regimen for the introduction or alteration of medication, how to deal with attacks, when and how to seek help and reference to specific advice such as that relating to driving. Reference could be included to items on the counselling checklist (Chapter 8, pages 110 and 111).

The main choice for treatment in a newly diagnosed patient is between sodium valproate and carbamazepine. The former has the widest spectrum of activity and is not contraindicated in any type of seizure, which favours its use in newly diagnosed epilepsy when the type of epilepsy is not yet clear. The main limitation of carbamazepine is that it is ineffective in absence attacks and myoclonus, although it may be slightly more effective in complex partial seizures. Slight differences in side-effects, especially in women, may indicate a preferred choice.

The process can perhaps be best understood by referring to case studies.

Case study 3

Jackie, referred to earlier (pages 35, 46), was considered to have partial epilepsy, and at 12 weeks into her pregnancy she was started on carbamazepine. She was started on a small dose of 200 mg each night for a week, and this was increased to 200 mg night and morning in the second week. A fortnight later, this was increased to 600 mg daily and she remained on that dose. Her pregnancy was uneventful, she had no further seizures over the next 2 years and decided to discontinue her medication, which she did successfully. An electroencephalogram (EEG), carried out during her pregnancy, showed a left temporal lobe focus, confirming the focal nature of her epilepsy.

Treatment failure

Although most patients will respond to treatment, a few will fall victim to side-effects; for others, control may not be achieved on the maximum tolerated dosage. The type of epilepsy or seizures may become clearer with time, either through investigations or in the expression of seizures. The need may arise to change to another drug, either another first-line drug if it is suitable or a second-line drug.

If seizures continue, both the diagnosis and compliance should be reviewed. Specialist advice on this and further drug manipulation is probably desirable, and the possibility of 'non-epileptic attacks' should be considered (see Chapter 4, pages 38–40 and Table 4.2, page 39).

If changing to an alternative first-line drug does not help, then two first-line drugs can be given together. If control does not improve, a second-line drug or one of the new add-on drugs may be tried.

The next case study shows a less straightforward series of events.

Case study 1

Margaret, aged 14 years, arrived home from school and was watching television when she experienced a tonic–clonic seizure. She was seen within a few weeks by a neurologist, who told her that she had epilepsy, and would have it all her life. She was not to swim, climb or ride a bicycle. He advised treatment with phenytoin 100 mg t.d.s., despite her having only one attack. After about 10 days, Margaret became ataxic and developed a rash, and so the phenytoin was stopped. She had a second tonic–clonic seizure shortly afterwards. An EEG taken by this time was normal. A second neurologist recommended sodium valproate; this was therefore started. There were no further seizures, but Margaret was distressed by thinning of her hair. Nevertheless, she continued with treatment, although she quietly dropped it down to 400 mg and later 200 mg daily. After 2 years without seizures, she stopped treatment and remained seizure-free until she took her first driving lesson at the age of 19 years, on which occasion she had a further tonic–clonic seizure. She resumed treatment with sodium valproate but took it in decreasing dosage, eventually discontinuing it a year later. She then had a further tonic–clonic seizure. On this occasion, she noticed that the attack had been preceded by a sensation of 'slowing down and going backwards', and later commented that she remembered having similar sensations before. It was concluded that her epilepsy was probably focal in origin and she agreed to go back on treatment. Because of the problems with hair thinning she was put on treatment with carbamazepine, and remained free from seizures while on this drug.

Comment

Margaret had the misfortune to develop reactions to the first two drugs. The sudden stopping of the phenytoin was unavoidable and may have precipitated the second tonic–clonic seizure. Disregarding the issue of treating after only one seizure, the phenytoin would have been better introduced more slowly, starting with 200 mg daily, and could have been given in a once daily dose. It was clear that Margaret took her medication as it suited her, but nevertheless she only had seizures when she stopped it altogether. As in Jackie's case, the focal nature of Margaret's epilepsy became clearer with time. Like most patients, she was adequately controlled on one drug. Treatment is, of course, about more than drugs, and the advice and information given by the first specialist was devastating, and wrong. Years later, Margaret, seizure-free, has a family, lives a normal life, drives a car and swims. She never really fancied rock climbing anyway.

Why review patients with chronic epilepsy?

It has been shown in general practice [12,13] that reviewing patients with epilepsy, reducing polypharmacy and changing treatment to achieve optimal benefit from anti-epileptic drugs can result in improved seizure control in 27% of patients. Side-effects, especially sedation, can be reduced in 24%, and general well-being improved.

Of the 12–15 patients with epilepsy on an average GP's list, most are likely to be well controlled. Seven or eight will continue to have seizures. Only a minority of three or four will have very frequent seizures. Treatment may be inappropriate or inadequate, some may be on polytherapy and suffering drug side-effects. Poor compliance may be the main underlying problem in those with poor control, and possibly a consequence of inadequate explanation and support. Even some who are seizure-free may be on polytherapy at an inappropriate dosage and suffer drug side-effects. Most patients may never have benefited from adequate explanations about their epilepsy or their treatment.

Understandably, even if they can find the time, not many GPs may feel confident enough to review patients with a view to changing from one drug to another. So why should review even be considered? First of all, most of the benefits to patients and families come from having an opportunity to ask questions and receive explanations. Where medication needs attention, this usually only involves adjusting existing medication and encouraging compliance. The few patients who need radical changes should probably have specialist review. It is important to anticipate that a possible consequence of taking an interest, and encouraging compliance in particular, is that of drug side-effects when they are actually taken 'as instructed'.

The process of reviewing patients with chronic epilepsy

Patients must of course be willing to be reviewed. It may seem unnecessary to state this, but invitations out of the blue, especially by post, offering to review a patient's epilepsy can backfire. Some patients simply prefer to be left alone, particularly if there is an implication that the doctor might want to change treatment. Not infrequently, the diagnosis has never been acknowledged as epilepsy, or if it has, it may have been concealed from a spouse. It is best to suggest a review when a prescription is due. Set aside at least half an hour, preferably longer; consider involving a practice nurse. Remember that you only have a dozen or so patients with epilepsy on your list, and that it is worthwhile.

• Start by defining the main problems as seen by the patient, for example, the severity and frequency of seizures, problems with drug side-effects and psychosocial problems. The latter may predominate, and assistance to obtain a disability living allowance may feature as being more important to someone with disabling epilepsy than aggressive attempts to improve control.

• Next, the correctness of the diagnosis should be checked as with a new patient. Seeking fresh descriptions of seizures will frequently cause surprise. A patient thought to have only tonic–clonic seizures preceded by an aura may be found to also experience complex partial seizures. Often, the seizure type or epilepsy syndrome will become clearer, and with this the appropriateness and adequacy of the current drug regimen and general advice and information.

• Ascertain the frequency and severity of *each* type of seizure experienced by the individual from the onset up to the present.

• Enquire about current anti-epileptic medication, dosage, how and when taken. Is it being taken as recommended, are there problems in remembering? Is it appropriate for the seizure type and for the particular patient? Enquire also about past anti-epileptic medication, whether it was effective or not, and why it was stopped.

• If a patient is seizure-free, the question of altering medication only arises if there are troublesome side-effects, or if there is a case for withdrawing treatment (see later).

• If a patient is still experiencing seizures, the most likely reason is poor compliance; the next is an inadequate dose of an appropriate anti-epileptic drug. Support and ingenuity in devising ways of remembering to take tablets will often prove effective (see Chapter 8, page 122). Specialist nurses, who are now employed in an increasing number of epilepsy services, have proved very effective in helping patients and families to achieve seizure control by tackling compliance. It may be that a practice nurse could undertake a similar role with equal success.

• Altering treatment becomes a consideration once compliance has been checked out, and if seizures are still a problem. Obviously, patients must be agreeable to having their treatment altered; some may prefer to leave well alone, particularly if they have encountered difficulties in the past. Occasional seizures may have come to be preferred to drug side-effects. If changing treatment is desirable, and other clinicians are involved with a patient, it will be necessary to consult or at least inform them. If the involvement relates specifically to the epilepsy, a joint plan is obviously desirable. Patients with chronic, poorly controlled seizures are best managed with specialist help, but some may not be willing to have it. Patients whose epilepsy relapses or worsens, or who are found to have developed new neurological symptoms or signs, require specialist review.

Altering treatment in the patient with chronic epilepsy

So, where it appears that a patient might benefit from alterations to treatment, a decision has to be made about whether there is a need for specialist advice. Some straightforward adjustments to treatment can be readily undertaken in general practice, for example, simplifying tablet-taking to a once or twice daily dose where this is possible, using slow-release preparations to facilitate this if necessary and optimizing the doses of anti-epileptic medication already being taken by a patient.

There is no reason why introducing a new anti-epileptic drug or changing drugs should not be undertaken by a GP, especially if the alternative is to do nothing where there is a problem in getting specialist advice, or because a patient is unwilling to be referred. The principles described earlier in starting treatment in a newly diagnosed patient (page 53) must be followed, particularly in regard to introducing new medication gradually, avoiding the reduction or withdrawal of existing anti-epileptic medication until the new drug has reached therapeutic levels and always avoiding sudden withdrawal.

There comes a point where it becomes advisable, or even essential, to have expert help. Obviously, if seizure control worsens or adding on drugs does not help, it is unwise to persist without help. Figure 5.1 outlines a structured approach to anti-epileptic treatment change.

The following case study shows how review can eventually benefit a patient.

Case study 2

Eileen, aged 42 years, started with epilepsy at the age of 13 years. Her seizures at first were tonic–clonic, and typically occurred when first rising in the morning. Occasionally, she had them at night. She had them more often if she was short of sleep. She also had what she called 'minor attacks'. In these, she was briefly unaware and stuttered. Over the years, she was treated with a range of drugs, phenobarbitone, phenytoin, clonazepam, carbamazepine and mysoline. At the age of 32 years, she moved and changed her doctor, who reviewed her epilepsy and her treatment. At this time, she was taking mysoline, phenytoin and carbamazepine, she complained of being tired all the time and having an awful memory. Her tonic–clonic fits occurred about once a month, her 'stuttering attacks' several times a week. It was concluded that she had partial epilepsy, and that her 'stuttering attacks' were complex partial seizures. Since phenytoin was the only drug that she was taking in a near therapeutic dose, it was agreed that, after increasing the latter, first mysoline and then carbamazepine would be withdrawn.

Very quickly, Eileen improved in her general well-being. Her tonic–clonic seizures became less frequent, but her 'stuttering attacks', which occurred mainly in the mornings, were only slightly improved. She was, however, happy with the improvement. She continued on monotherapy on maximum dosage of phenytoin for several years, but then developed a rare complication of phenytoin therapy, peripheral neuropathy. She was referred to a neurologist who changed her treatment to carbamazepine. Eileen's 'stuttering attacks' then became much worse; if in the kitchen or at table, crockery she was handling would go flying. It became apparent that she was experiencing myoclonic seizures, not complex partial seizures. Eileen had juvenile myoclonic epilepsy, and her treatment was changed to sodium valproate with good results.

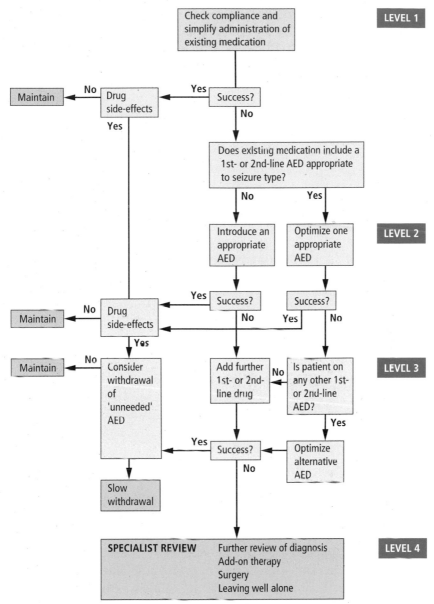

Fig. 5.1 Chronic epilepsy: a structured approach to treatment change. AED, anti-epileptic drug.

Comment

The opportunity for the first review came when Eileen registered with a new doctor and change of treatment was moderately successful, even though the diagnosis of juvenile myoclonic epilepsy was missed, as it often was until recently. Although changing to carbamazepine made matters worse, it did so only briefly and drew attention to the correct diagnosis and control of her seizures after many years.

Continuing management

Good continuing care and management, in addition to providing prescriptions, involves being available and able to answer questions and to respond to changing needs. The nature and expression of the epilepsy itself may change for an individual, as well as circumstances such as growing up, growing old or becoming pregnant. One individual's epilepsy may worsen, most will remain well controlled, another will come off treatment altogether and remain well.

The extremes of status epilepticus and of being able to come off treatment altogether are covered below. Providing care in special circumstances, such as childhood, in the elderly or pregnancy, is covered in Chapter 8.

Status epilepticus

Status epilepticus is a medical emergency with a significant morbidity and mortality, and requires urgent hospital admission. Patients and relatives should be advised to send for an ambulance if a convulsive seizure persists or recurrence goes on for 10 minutes or more. If a doctor is present, intravenous or rectal diazepam should be administered in a dose of 10–20 mg. The rectal route is less likely to cause apnoea than the intravenous route. Intramuscular or oral diazepam are useless. Midazolam has recently been found to have advantages over diazepam in emergency use, since it can be given intranasally or by buccal installation. There is no conveniently marketed device for installation and it is given in a dose of 10 mg drawn up in a syringe.

Tonic–clonic attacks occurring close together with or without brief recovery between seizures should lead to urgent hospital admission.

Stopping treatment

The question of stopping treatment is likely to arise after a period free from seizures. Certainly, most individuals are keen to know when, if ever, they will be able to stop treatment with the possibility of remaining free from seizures. It is easier to come to a decision with children, since withdrawal is more often successful, and the risk of losing a driving licence or a job has not yet arisen. In most children who have been seizure-free for 2 years or more, drugs can be withdrawn over 2–3 months (2 years after stopping treatment, 75% will be seizure-free).

Withdrawal in adults is more problematic. One study shows 59% are seizure-free 2 years after slow withdrawal. Most adults, understandably, are unwilling to risk seizure recurrence, with their subsequent consequences for employment and driving.

If a decision is taken to stop treatment, it should be carried out over many weeks or months, one drug at a time. Those who have experienced few seizures do best, and those with complex partial seizures are more likely to relapse. **With some epileptic syndromes (e.g. juvenile myoclonic epilepsy), withdrawal should not be attempted.**

Interestingly, many patients with mild epilepsy, and those who have had few seizures, appear to simply leave off slowly of their own accord.

Care plans

Among the principles of treatment in new patients is the importance of having a care plan for the patient. This should include instructions for changing treatment and specific advice about matters relevant to the patient. Care plans are useful aids in managing complicated treatment changes and long-term care for individuals. They are also valuable for the overall organization of planned care for chronic disease management for all patients with a particular problem. Care plans are dealt with more fully in Chapter 9.

Surgery and other treatment

Despite the good prognosis for the control of epilepsy with anti-epileptic drugs for most patients, a minority continue to have seizures. For some of these, surgery is now a realistic alternative. Behavioural therapy, including biofeedback and very recently vagal nerve stimulation, appear to be effective in some cases. Other treatments, variously described as 'alternative' or 'complementary' treatments, for which claims are made include relaxation therapy, aromatherapy, acupuncture and homeopathy.

Surgical treatment

A concise, but comprehensive, review of surgery for epilepsy can be found in *Epilepsy* by Appleton *et al.* [48].

Surgical treatment has a long history, but few operations have been carried out until relatively recently. Recently, due to advances in presurgical investigations and operative techniques, there has been a rapid increase in the number of centres offering surgery and in the number of operations performed. Results are encouraging. In the 5-year period ending in 1990, 2429 operations for anterior temporal lobectomy resulted in 67.9% becoming seizure-free and a further 24% improved. The results for amygdalohippocampectomy were similar. Overall mortality is less than 1%, and morbidity due to operation in the form of hemianopia and hemiplegia is 3–4%.

Types of operation

A range of procedures are now carried out. Basically, they are divided into two kinds: resections of epileptogenic or structurally abnormal tissue, which are intended to be curative, and functional palliative procedures which consist of disconnecting epileptogenic cortical foci from the rest of the brain.

The most common cause of refractory partial seizures is an epileptogenic focus in the temporal lobe, and two-thirds of all operations for epilepsy involve resections of the temporal lobe. Fortunately, seizures emanating from the temporal lobe are easier to lateralize than from other parts of the cortex, and the removal of the temporal lobe is tolerated well compared with the occipital, parietal or frontal lobes.

The work-up for surgery

Any patient with partial seizures who fails to benefit from optimum treatment with anti-epileptic drugs can be considered for surgery. It usually takes at least 2 years to reach this point, having worked through all the possible drug regimes. Presurgical evaluation can be quite formidable and includes the following criteria.

1 The patient must be able to benefit from cure. So epilepsy must be the main disability. A low IQ, e.g. less than 70, would be a poor starting point, because of the possibility of further loss of function as a consequence of surgery. Age must be usually less than 50 years (most operations are carried out on patients in the second decade). The patient must have the emotional resources to go through it all.

2 An epileptogenic focus must be definable by imaging and/or by EEG localization. Magnetic resonance imaging (MRI) has superseded computed tomography (CT) scanning and is the most important and effective imaging technique. Other techniques used include positron emission tomography (PET) and single proton emission computed tomography (SPECT). These identify changes in blood flow and metabolism in relation to ictal events and are mainly of confirmatory value.

The EEG is the main tool in localizing epileptic foci. Some of the special electrodes used are invasive. Foramen ovale and sphenoidal electrodes are used to lateralize seizures from the medial aspect of the temporal lobes and subdural or depth electrodes may be used to define foci elsewhere.

3 It must be established that postoperative cerebral functioning will be acceptable. Basically, this amounts to assessing the importance of what the side that is to be resected does. Can it be removed without the risk of much loss of cerebral function?

The evaluation consists of tests of intellect and memory and tests to localize function. The intracarotid amytal test (Wada test) is used to establish whether the temporal lobe on the opposite side to the proposed resection can sustain memory afterwards. It is somewhat invasive. The test involves passing a cannula into a femoral artery and on into the carotid. A short-acting barbiturate is injected which produces hemiparesis and dysphasia for language. Memory testing is carried out before, during and afterwards. Confirmation of language lateralization and memory function is established by presenting information during anaesthesia and assessing remaining memory afterwards.

Gamma knife surgery

Radiosurgery involves the delivery of high doses of radiation to carefully targeted areas, and is only used if a focus can be identified very precisely, which is not often possible. In gamma knife surgery, 201 separate rays are focused through a helmet-like hemisphere held in a stereotactic frame over the patient's head. Most are treated as day cases; treatment planning takes one to one and a half hours, and the treatment itself around 20 minutes. Although the treatment is still in a research stage, 70–75% of patients are reported to benefit [49]. About 10–15% become seizure free, and the treatment usually reduces the severity and frequency of seizures. There are no recorded cases of a patient's condition getting worse as a result of this treatment.

Vagal nerve stimulation

This uses a device which has been developed to stimulate the vagal nerve in order to control seizures. The mode of action is uncertain, but since mental and physical activity decreases the chance of a seizure, it is speculated that vagal stimulation activates the brain and inhibits the development of a seizure. Early results from Bristol [50] show gradual benefit with optimum results after 18 months to 2 years. Some 70% of patients secure some reduction in seizure frequency; the majority report improvement in the nature of their seizures—shorter, less severe, quicker recovery and improved quality of life.

Implantation is relatively simple. The device is placed within the chest with a stimulating lead connected to the vagus nerve in the neck. In addition to programmed stimulation, the patient can start stimulation by means of a magnet, if he or she feels a seizure starting.

Behavioural therapy and biofeedback

The background to this is the evidence that children can both inhibit and induce seizures, and that many adults are known to develop behavioural strategies to inhibit or stop the spread of their seizures.

Studying events around the time of seizures helps to define those aspects of a patient's emotional life or behaviour that will trigger or inhibit seizure activity. This provides a basis for an individual to control his or her epilepsy.

Using a behavioural approach together with EEG biofeedback has been shown to result in individuals achieving improved control, when they had previously been resistant to anti-epileptic drugs. Most of this work has been carried out overseas. There have been no randomized trials.

Seizure alert dogs

It seems that dogs can be trained to recognize specific changes preceding a seizure in humans [51] and to signal a warning to the owner, giving enough time to take control of the situation. The numbers so far are small, but it seems that the dogs can give as much as 15–45 minutes' warning. Unexpectedly, patients have found seizure frequency to be reduced. It is thought that increased predictability enabled the subjects to engage in more everyday activities with greater confidence. It is known that being occupied can reduce seizure frequency.

Aromatherapy

Interestingly, of so-called 'alternative' and 'complementary' treatments, aromatherapy does seem to benefit some individuals with epilepsy, although there have been no randomized trials. The relaxing and calming oils relieve tension and stress, which are known to precipitate seizures. On the other hand, some oils are reputed to have the potential to trigger seizures. Aromatherapy has been used and evaluated by Dr T. Betts and his team in the Neuropsychiatry and Seizure Clinic at Queen Elizabeth Psychiatric Hospital, Birmingham. Oils that may be helpful include ylang-ylang, camomile and lavender. Oils to avoid are rosemary, hyssop, sweet fennel and sage.

Any patient contemplating aromatherapy should contact a trained aromatherapist, but should keep on taking the tablets. The International Federation of Aromatherapists, The Royal Masonic Hospital, London W6 0TN, may help find an approved therapist.

6 Treatment: Individual Anti-Epileptic Drug Profiles

This chapter provides basic information on the important anti-epileptic drugs. Fuller information can be found in the *British National Formulary*, individual data sheets, *Prescribers Notes* and *Drug and Therapeutics Bulletins*. For a full recent description, see *Handbook of Epilepsy Treatment* [52].

First-line drugs

Carbamazepine (Tegretol)

Carbamazepine has become established as the major first-line anti-epileptic drug for partial, and some generalized, seizures. It is a highly effective and usually well tolerated drug. However, if side-effects are a problem, a slow-release preparation (Tegretol Retard) is available. Since swings in serum levels are much reduced in the slow-release form, side-effects are fewer and effects on the developing foetus are theoretically fewer. For these reasons, many specialists use the slow-release preparation routinely.

Indications

The primary indications for carbamazepine are as a first-line or add-on therapy for partial or generalized seizures (excluding absence and myoclonus). It is also indicated in Lennox–Gastaut and other childhood epilepsy syndromes. It may make the myoclonus of juvenile myoclonic epilepsy worse.

Therapeutic use

Sudden introduction of carbamazepine is liable to cause side-effects, especially nausea and vomiting in the first week. Carbamazepine as an enzyme inducer increases the metabolism not only of some other drugs, but also of itself. Over the first 2 or 3 weeks of use, its half-life drops from 25–45 hours to 8–24 hours.

Introduction in a small dose is therefore best, although 200 mg at night in the first week is tolerated by most adults. If there is no urgency, 100 mg in the first week followed by 200 mg in the second week may be better. After this, the dose may be increased to 200 mg b.d. and a fortnight later to 300 mg b.d. Thereafter, if seizures recur, the dose may be increased by 200 mg in monthly increments. Most adults will be controlled on 600–1200 mg/day, but some will require and tolerate 1600–2000 mg. A twice-daily dose is usually adequate.

The standard preparation can be effective in twice-daily dosage, but often needs to be taken three times a day. If compliance is a problem, or if side-effects occur, the long-acting Retard formulation should be tried.

Note: If tablets of Tegretol Retard have to be split, they should be used within 24 hours. It is inadvisable to mix the preparations.

Oxcarbazepine, recently introduced, is closely related to carbamazepine and is a useful substitute for patients already controlled on carbamazepine who become intolerant or hypersensitive to it. Sometimes, when added to carbamazepine, it has an additive effect (see oxcarbazepine below).

Side-effects

Common central nervous system (CNS) side-effects include sedation, blurred vision, diplopia, being off-balance, headache and drowsiness. A slow increase in dose can help avoid these effects, but sometimes it is necessary to spread the daily dose or take the slow-release formulation. Carbamazepine causes rash in 5–10% of patients; if rashes are very mild and transient, it is not always necessary to stop the drug. Leucopenia and hyponatraemia occur but are usually not clinically important. In common with other anti-epileptics, carbamazepine has some teratogenic effects, in particular a slight increase in the risk of spina bifida (1%) when taken by women during pregnancy. Despite this, carbamazepine is the drug considered safest in pregnancy for those with partial and secondarily generalized epilepsy.

Interactions

Important interactions are mainly due to liver enzyme induction.
• The drug speeds its own metabolism and that of phenobarbitone, sodium valproate and lamotrigine, and also of the oral contraceptive pill, theophylline and warfarin.
• Lamotrigine may precipitate carbamazepine toxicity.

- Erythromycin, dextropropoxyphene (Co-proxamol) and omeprazole (Losec) all raise carbamazepine levels.

Sodium valproate (Epilim)

Sodium valproate is mainly used in an enteric-coated formulation, but recently a controlled-release preparation has been introduced (Epilim Chrono). Most patients are controlled on a twice-daily dose of the normal preparation, and the main advantage of the slow-release preparation appears to lie in reducing swings in serum levels, which may be a cause of side-effects and are particularly undesirable in pregnancy. Epilim Chrono is now licensed for once-daily dosage.

Indications

Sodium valproate is effective against both generalized and partial seizures. It is the only first-line drug to be effective against petit mal absence. **It is the drug of choice for patients with primary generalized epilepsy suffering from tonic–clonic attacks and/or petit mal absences and juvenile myoclonic epilepsy.** It is a broad-spectrum drug which does not exacerbate any seizures.

Therapeutic use

Sodium valproate is very straightforward to introduce. Nowadays, the manufacturer recommends that adults have a starting dose of 600 mg/day, increasing in 200 mg increments every 3 days up to 1500–2500 mg/day. Some specialists start with 500 mg, increasing by 500 mg increments. It really depends upon the severity of the situation, and rapid escalation of the larger dose is more appropriate when dealing with changes in therapy in chronic, poorly controlled epilepsy. It is reasonable for most newly diagnosed patients to commence with 400–600 mg/day. If further seizures occur above 600 mg, then 200 mg in weekly increments is suggested (weekly increments are easier for patients to remember). Most adults will require 600–1500 mg. Twice-daily dosage is usually adequate, but it may need to be taken three times daily, or alternatively, the long-acting preparation, Epilim Chrono, may be used. The latter is available in 500, 300 and 200 mg tablets and may be given once daily. The manufacturers state that it may be switched to directly from the standard preparation, without loss of seizure control. Routine serum level monitoring of sodium valproate is pointless unless poor compliance is suspected.

Side-effects

Although sodium valproate can cause sedation in some, it is generally well tolerated. A few patients suffer gastrointestinal side-effects, heartburn, nausea and vomiting, not always avoided by enteric-coated preparations. Hair loss and rashes occur, but relatively infrequently. Hair loss tends to be transient and recovers after withdrawal, but regrowth may be curly. Weight gain is fairly common and can be a problem for teenage girls and young women. Tremor can occur at higher doses. Hepatotoxicity has been reported, but is very rare and has only affected very young children with learning disability.

There are important considerations when prescribing for females of reproductive age. In common with other major anti-epileptics, there is a slightly increased incidence of foetal abnormality. Spina bifida has been reported in 1–1.5%, but usually this is associated with high dosage and polytherapy with other anti-epileptics (see Chapter 7 on epilepsy and pregnancy). Valproate can also have endocrine effects, with alterations in sex hormone levels, resulting in anovulatory cycles, amenorrhoea and polycystic ovary syndrome [53].

Interactions

Valproate given with phenytoin can lead to low serum levels of the latter in the presence of high-tissue levels and even toxicity. The metabolism of lamotrigine is reduced by valproate and should be given in reduced dosage when prescribed with valproate (see later). Other drugs can affect valproate levels; phenytoin, phenobarbitone and carbamazepine can reduce levels; antacids reduce absorption; and naproxen and salicylates displace valproate from albumin-binding and raise levels.

Second-line drugs

Oxcarbazepine (Trileptal)

This drug has only recently been licensed in the UK but has been used extensively abroad since the 1980s, and is considered to be a first-line therapy in some countries. It shares many characteristics with carbamazepine, but is easier to introduce and has fewer side-effects or drug interactions—an important interaction being with the contraceptive pill. It may prove to be an easy drug to use in general practice.

Indications

The primary indications are as add-on or monotherapy in partial and secondarily generalized seizures. In general, its indications are the same as those for carbamazepine. It is similar in efficacy to carbamazepine, phenytoin and valproate. It is a useful substitute for patients already controlled on carbamazepine who become intolerant or hypersensitive to it. Sometimes, when added to carbamazepine, it has an additive effect.

Therapeutic use

It can be introduced more quickly than carbamazepine. In adults, a starting dose of 600 mg per day can be increased weekly in 600 mg increments to a maintenance dose of between 900 mg and 2400 mg per day, in a twice-daily dosage. Most patients require 900–1200 mg per day. Children should be started on 10 mg/kg per day, increasing in 10 mg/kg steps up to 30 mg/kg per day.

It is said [52] that in substituting oxcarbazepine for carbamazepine there is no need to titrate up the newer drug and then titrate down the other. Substitution at a carbamazepine : oxcarbazepine ratio of 200 : 300 can be carried out abruptly.

Side-effects

The side-effects are very similar to those of carbamazepine but are less frequent or severe. Oxcarbazepine's side-effect profile is better than that of carbamazepine, phenytoin or valproate. Of adverse effects, skin rash is relatively common—in about 5% of patients. The rash is similar to that caused by carbamazepine, but having a rash with the latter does not mean that a change to oxcarbazepine will lead to a rash (only 25% risk). The most common dose-related side-effects are tiredness, headache, dizziness and ataxia. Other side-effects include weight gain, alopecia, nausea and gastrointestinal disturbance. Hyponatraemia, as with carbamazepine, is common but usually asymptomatic or mild, and not of clinical importance except in patients taking diuretics or the elderly. Excessive fluid intake, e.g. large quantities of beer, should be avoided.

Interactions

Oxcarbazepine has less liver enzyme induction than carbamazepine and has fewer interactions. The most important is that with hormonal contraceptives. Although oxcarbazepine does not alter the levels of other anti-epileptic drugs, the enzyme-inducing effects of carbamazepine, phenytoin and phenobarbitone can reduce the bioavailability of the effective metabolite of oxcarbazepine (MHD). In short, patients co-medicated with any of these drugs may need a higher dose of oxcarbazepine.

There is insufficient evidence about safety in pregnancy, and the drug should not, as yet, be prescribed in pregnancy or lactation.

Lamotrigine (Lamictal)

Indications

Lamotrigine was introduced in 1991. It is an effective add-on therapy for partial and secondarily generalized seizures. It is also effective in absence, myoclonic, tonic, clonic and tonic–clonic seizures, and therapy-resistant Lennox–Gastaut syndrome (see Chapter 7). Lamotrigine was licensed for monotherapy in 1995 with potential as a first-line drug.

Therapeutic use

The starting dose depends on current treatment. Slow introduction reduces the risk of rash.

Monotherapy comprises 25 mg/day for 2 weeks, then 50 mg/day for 2 weeks, then increasing in monthly steps to a maintenance dose of 100–200 mg/day either in a single or divided dose. (A few patients may go up to 500 mg/day.)

For patients on sodium valproate, 25 mg is given on alternate days for 2 weeks, then 25 mg/day for 2 weeks, then increasing in monthly steps to a maintenance dose of 50–100 mg twice daily.

For patients on other anti-epileptic drugs, 50 mg/day is increased after 2 weeks to 50 mg twice daily for 2 weeks, and then by 100 mg monthly as necessary up to a maintenance dose of 200 mg twice daily.

Side-effects

Headache, nausea and vomiting, diplopia, dizziness and ataxia are most common. A skin rash, usually maculopapular, occurs in 5%, early in treatment. The risk of this may be reduced by slow introduction. Rare toxic reactions include rash plus malaise, fever, arthralgia, myalgia and lymphadenopathy. A few develop erythema multiforme and Stevens–Johnson syndrome.

Interactions

Patients taking carbamazepine may develop neurotoxic side-effects after the introduction of lamotrigine. These disappear after reduction of either drug.

Sodium valproate inhibits the metabolism of lamotrigine, doubling its half-life and reducing the dose of lamotrigine needed. Conversely, enzyme-inducing drugs such as carbamazepine, phenytoin and phenobarbitone accelerate the metabolism of lamotrigine, reducing its half-life by 50% and necessitating a larger dose of lamotrigine.

Phenytoin (Epanutin)

Now falling out of use as a first-line drug by most specialists because of its side-effects and difficulty in use, phenytoin is still popular among some because it can be given in a once-daily dose.

Indications

Phenytoin is effective in tonic–clonic, simple and complex partial seizures.

Therapeutic use

Phenytoin is a very effective drug which can be difficult to use because dose requirements can vary greatly between individuals. Start with 200 mg o.n. Do not normally adjust more than once a month. **The therapeutic range is so small that a small increase in dose can take a patient to toxic levels**, e.g. once a dose of 300 mg/day has been reached, 25 mg increments only should be considered. Phenytoin, despite its disadvantages, suits many patients and since it has a long half-life can be given as a single daily dose.

A few patients require high dosage, e.g. over 500 mg. Low serum levels are usually associated with poor or erratic compliance. **A pep talk combined with an increase in dose can easily lead to toxicity, so beware**.

Side-effects

Phenytoin has similar toxic side-effects to carbamazepine, i.e. vertigo, diplopia, ataxia and headache. Sedation and depression of mental functioning are more of a problem than with carbamazepine. Rashes and swelling of lymph nodes can occur. Other important side-effects are associated with long-term use and include those affecting appearance, coarsening of features, acne-like rash and gum hyperplasia. Rare idiosyncratic effects include macrocytosis, liver damage and peripheral neuropathy. If signs of toxicity are evident, serum levels should be checked.

Interactions

Phenytoin, in common with carbamazepine, interacts with other anti-epileptics by increasing liver metabolism. Both interfere with warfarin and the contraceptive pill and omeprazole (Losec). Sodium valproate can cause toxicity in the presence of apparently normal serum levels. Vigabatrin can result in a fall in phenytoin levels of 20% after 4 weeks.

Phenobarbitone/primidone (Mysoline)

A very effective but sedative drug. Withdrawal can lead to withdrawal seizures. For practical purposes, phenobarbitone and primidone can be regarded as the same drug, since primidone is broken down to phenobarbitone.

Indications

Effective in tonic–clonic, clonic and partial seizures.

Therapeutic use

Dose up to 200 mg/day in two or three divided doses. The drug is prone to lead to withdrawal seizures after chronic use.

Side-effects

Rashes. Sedation is common and a serious problem, and behavioural disturbances are caused in children. Phenobarbitone is effective and cheap and therefore important worldwide, but because of its side-effects and greater toxicity is prescribed less frequently in the developed world. It is only used as a last resort in patients who cannot tolerate other drugs.

Interactions

Phenobarbitone is an enzyme inducer which can influence the metabolism of many drugs, including oral contraceptives, other anti-epileptics, warfarin and thyroxine.

Add-on drugs

Vigabatrin (Sabril)

Vigabatrin is a powerful drug with specific indications, but beset with serious side-effects, particularly psychiatric and visual, which limit its use.

Indications

Vigabatrin was introduced in 1989 as an add-on drug for partial and secondarily generalized seizures. It has proved to be particularly effective against refractory complex partial seizures, but less so with secondary generalization. It is not so effective against primary generalized epilepsy, and can make myoclonic epilepsy and absence worse. It is effective against infantile spasms, for which it is the drug of choice despite its other disadvantages, and also Lennox–Gastaut syndrome.

Therapeutic use

Treatment in adults should start with 500 mg once or twice daily to allow tolerance to sedation and to anticipate behavioural side-effects. The drug should be withdrawn immediately if there is agitation or thought disorder. Thereafter, the dose should be increased by 250–500 mg increments every 1–2 weeks. The average maintenance dose is 1000–2000 mg, although 25% will require 3000 mg. In children, the starting dose is 40 mg/kg daily with maintenance doses of 80–100 mg/kg daily usual. Lower doses should be used in renal impairment, and withdrawal should be done slowly, e.g. 500 mg increments fortnightly in adults.

Side-effects

Minor side-effects are common and include fatigue, drowsiness, headache, dizziness, weight increase, tremor and double vision. More serious are neuropsychiatric adverse events, notably depression (5%), agitation (7%), confusion, and occasionally psychosis.

Also of concern is the mounting evidence of serious peripheral visual defects. These are asymptomatic until the late stages, and only 10% of patients notice. Clinical visual field testing by confrontation does not pick it up, and examination with either the Goldmann perimetry, or the computerized Humphrey field analyser, is necessary. The prevalence in adults has been reported at 30% [54]. The manufacturer reports a prevalence of 10–20% [55] and recommends six-monthly visual field assessments. In its recently revised guideline [56], the Vigabatrin Paediatric Advisory Group recommends visual field testing before prescribing vigabatrin and six-monthly checks thereafter.

Interactions

Vigabatrin produces a fall of about 20% in serum phenytoin after around 4 weeks, and may therefore require a small increase in phenytoin dosage at this stage.

Gabapentin (Neurontin)

Indications

Gabapentin is a useful drug for the add-on treatment of partial or secondarily generalized seizures, for which it appears to be effective. Its lack of interactions makes it attractive, and it is useful in cases where renal or hepatic disease is present. It is, however, ineffective in most generalized seizure disorders and in myoclonus. Overall, gabapentin has modest efficacy, particularly at lower doses, and is not usually effective in severe epilepsy.

Therapeutic use

The drug has a short half-life and therefore has to be taken three times daily. The manufacturers recommend 300 mg on day 1, two doses of 300 mg on day 2, three doses of 300 mg on day 3, up to 1200 mg/day. The dose can be increased to a maximum of 3600 mg/day in three divided doses. Patients with refractory epilepsy often require 2400–4800 mg daily.

Side-effects and interactions

These are few, mainly somnolence, dizziness and ataxia, and are more prominent at higher doses. Gabapentin is not teratogenic in animals and does not interfere with other anti-epileptic drugs or oral contraceptives. Antacids reduce its bioavailability by 20%.

Topiramate (Topamax)

Indications

Topiramate is a powerful new anti-epileptic drug with a wide spectrum of anti-epileptic activity, but it has a high rate of side-effects. Initially introduced as add-on therapy in refractory partial epilepsy, with or without secondary generalization, it has been found to be effective in generalized epilepsy—tonic–clonic seizures, typical absence and myoclonus. It has proved effective as monotherapy in partial epilepsy, and is effective in children, including the Lennox–Gastaut syndrome.

Therapeutic use

Topiramate is given twice daily and should be introduced slowly to reduce the risk of side-effects. In adults, an initial dose of 25 mg daily can be increased fortnightly to 50 mg then 100 mg, after which fortnightly increments to a maintenance dose of 200–600 mg daily. Higher doses may be needed when combined with the enzyme-inducing drugs carbamazepine and phenytoin. The paediatric dose has not been fully defined, but the usual starting dose is 0.5–1 mg/kg daily, increased in 0.5–1 mg/kg increments fortnightly.

Side-effects

Adverse effects are a problem in 15% of patients and include ataxia, poor concentration, confusion, dizziness, fatigue, peripheral paraesthesiae, somnolence, disturbance of memory, depression, agitation and slowness of speech. Side-effects are less common in monotherapy. Many side-effects lessen after a few weeks if the drug is continued, and frequency and severity are less if doses are slowly titrated. The drug is better tolerated by children.

Weight loss can be considerable, especially in those overweight to begin with. There is also a risk of renal calculi.

Interactions

Phenytoin and carbamazepine induce topiramate's metabolism, dropping serum levels by 40–50%. Topiramate itself induces the metabolism of the oestrogenic component of the contraceptive pill, necessitating the use of a preparation containing at least 35 μg ethinyloestradiol.

Tiagabine (Gabitril)

Indications

Tiagabine was introduced as add-on therapy for refractory partial and secondarily generalized seizures. There is still only limited information about its efficacy in monotherapy. Its role in clinical practice is not yet clear. Tiagabine levels are lowered by co-medication with enzyme-inducing drugs.

Therapeutic use

Tiagabine should be taken with food to avoid high peak concentrations. In adults already on enzyme-inducing drugs, tiagabine should be introduced at a dose of 15 mg per day followed by weekly increments of 5–15 mg. The recommended oral maintenance daily dose for patients on enzyme-inducing drugs is 30–45 mg per day and 15–30 mg for those who are not. If there is a history of behavioural problems or depression, the drug should be introduced slowly under close supervision. It should not be used in pregnancy or during lactation and is contraindicated in severe hepatic impairment.

Side-effects

CNS side-effects are the most common and include dizziness, asthenia, nervousness, tremor, depression and emotional lability.

In view of the problems of loss of vision with vigabatrin, with which tiagabine has similarities, studies have been carried out to investigate any effect of this sort– so far none have been reported.

Interactions

Tiagabine does not itself induce enzyme activity, but its metabolism is markedly changed by co-administration of enzyme-inducing drugs such as carbamazepine and phenytoin.

Levetiracetam (Keppra) [52]

This is a highly effective new anti-epileptic drug, about to be licensed in the UK, with a good acceptability and low side-effect profile so far. It was first investigated in the 1980s for cognitive enhancement and anxiolytic properties and was found to have anti-epileptic properties. In early trials, it was found to have a powerful anti-epileptic effect against all types of partial seizures as add-on therapy, and later to be effective as monotherapy. It is effective in photosensitive epilepsy, myoclonic jerks, and juvenile myoclonic epilepsy refractory to valproate or lamotrigine.

Indications

Levetiracetam is currently licensed as add-on therapy in partial seizures with or without secondary generalization.

Therapeutic use

The starting dose is 500 mg twice daily followed by weekly increments of 500–1000 mg daily to a total of 3000 mg. The recommended range is 1000–3000 mg daily, but can be increased to 4000 mg. Caution is necessary in renal impairment or the elderly, where the dose should be lower.

Side-effects and interactions

Most side-effects are mild and include somnolence, asthenia, infection and dizziness. No significant interactions have been identified.

Clobazam (Frisium)

Indications

The main indication is as add-on therapy for partial and generalized seizures. It is also useful as intermittent therapy for short-term use, e.g. catamenial epilepsy and one-off prophylaxis for examinations, interviews or travel. It has value in non-convulsive status epilepticus.

It is a very effective add-on anti-epileptic for some patients resistant to first-line therapy. Clobazam is better tolerated than other benzodiazepines but is subject to the same disadvantage of development of tolerance in as many as 50% of patients within weeks or months.

Therapeutic use

The dosage is simple. In adults 10–30 mg daily, usually taken at night, or twice daily in a divided dose. Children aged 3–12 require up to half the adult dose. When prescribed for epilepsy in the UK, 'SLS' must be written on the prescription.

Side-effects and interactions

Side-effects are as for other benzodiazepines: sedation, dizziness, ataxia, blurred vision, occasionally behavioural disturbance, irritability, depression and loss of inhibition. There are few interactions; those with other anti-epileptic drugs are minor and not significant in clinical practice.

Other benzodiazepines

Diazepam (Valium) is effective when given intravenously or rectally in a dose of 5–10 mg in emergencies, but otherwise has little effect by other routes, e.g. intramuscularly. It may cause apnoea if given intravenously.

Midazolam has recently been found to have advantages over diazepam in emergency use, since it can be given intranasally or by buccal installation. There is no conveniently marketed device for installation and it is given in a dose of 10 mg drawn up in a syringe.

Clonazepam (Rivotril) has an anti-epileptic effect both parenterally in emergencies and orally for routine control, but long-term use is often associated with behavioural side-effects. In common with other benzodiazepines, tolerance may develop and it may cease to be effective.

Other drugs

Ethosuximide (Emeside, Zarontin)

Indications

Ethosuximide is a first-line or add-on therapy for generalized absence (petit mal) seizures. Its effects can be remarkable. It is equal in effect to valproate, which has largely replaced it because of valproate's additional effectiveness against tonic–clonic seizures.

Therapeutic use

In adults it is usual to start with 250 mg daily, increasing fortnightly by 250–500 mg to a maintenance dose of between 750 mg and 2000 mg in two divided doses. Children should start with 10–15 mg/kg daily, with incremental rises up to 20–40 mg/kg daily given in two or three divided doses. Plasma levels are useful; the target range is 300–700 µmol/L.

Side-effects

Ethosuximide has dose-related gastrointestinal side-effects which can be reduced by divided doses. Other side-effects include headache, sedation, behavioural change, irritability, depression, anxiety, and rarely a psychotic reaction. It should be used with caution if there is a psychiatric history.

Idiosyncratic reactions include skin rashes, which can be severe—erythema multiforme and Stevens–Johnson syndrome. Blood dyscrasias, systemic lupus erythematosis, pericarditis, myocarditis and thyroiditis.

Interactions

Ethosuximide does not affect the serum levels of other drugs, but valproate can increase ethosuximide by 50%, and hepatic enzyme-inducing drugs can reduce ethosuximide levels.

Piracetam (Nootropil)

Piracetam was originally developed as a possible memory-enhancing drug in the 1960s, 10 years later it was noticed to be effective in myoclonus, and has since been found to have remarkable effectiveness in cortical myoclonus from differing causes.

Indications

In epilepsy it is only indicated for myoclonus, usually as add-on therapy to valproate or benzodiazepines.

Therapeutic use

The initial dose is 7.2 g daily, then is rapidly increased by 4.8 g every 3 days up to 24 g daily, sometimes 32 g. Even when given in two or three divided doses, the bulk of tablets can be a problem.

Lower dosage is indicated in severe renal disease, and the drug is contra-indicated if the creatinine clearance is below 20 mL/min.

There is no published experience in children. Withdrawal needs to be gradual, as sudden withdrawal can cause severe myoclonus.

Side-effects and interactions

Apart from the difficulties with its bulk, this is a well-tolerated drug with a low incidence of side-effects. Reported side-effects include dizziness, insomnia, nausea and gastrointestinal discomfort, hyperkinesis, weight gain, drowsiness, tremulousness and agitation. Rash occurs in less than 1% of patients. No interactions have been identified.

Acetazolamide (Diamox)

Indications

Acetazolamide has been found to be effective in many seizure types. It can be effective as monotherapy in tonic–clonic seizures, in juvenile myoclonic epilepsy, in absences and as an add-on drug for partial epilepsy. It can be useful in catamenial epilepsy, starting with treatment 8–10 days before menstruation is due and continued for up to 10 days.

Therapeutic use

The usual dose is 250 mg one or three times daily. Tolerance often develops over 3–6 months, and a period of drug withdrawal will restore its efficacy.

Side-effects and interactions

Side-effects are mild and transient, and include lethargy, paraesthesiae, anorexia, headache, nausea, diarrhoea and visual changes. Acetazolamide has carbonic anhydrase activity, which can cause renal calculi to develop. Drug interactions are rare.

7 Epilepsy and the Individual: Epilepsy in Children and Adolescents, in Women, in Learning Disability and in the Elderly

The general approach to diagnosis, treatment and advice introduced in earlier chapters is not always exactly applicable or appropriate for every patient in all circumstances. The causes and presentation of epilepsy can be different at different ages. For example, the rarer epilepsy syndromes and primary generalized epilepsies are a feature of childhood, whereas most epilepsy in the elderly is localization-based. Causes of disturbed consciousness, other than epilepsy, and important in the differential diagnosis, can be different in the very young and the old.

Epilepsy in women can pose special problems, for example, increased seizure activity in relation to menstruation, the effects of some anti-epileptic drugs on contraception and the developing foetus, and epilepsy in pregnancy.

Treatment may have different implications for children, the elderly, those with learning disability, or women of childbearing age. This chapter deals with particular issues of epilepsy management in childhood, adolescence, learning disability, women and the elderly.

Epilepsy in childhood and adolescence

Seizures are common in infancy and early childhood. They are very frightening to parents, who may fear that their child is dying or destined to be brain damaged. As many as 5–6% of children experience attacks of altered consciousness at some time. However, most of these attacks and most convulsive attacks are *not* due to epilepsy, and misdiagnosis is a serious problem. The actual prevalence of epilepsy in children is about 4 per 1000 of the population.

Differences in epilepsy between children and adults

Children are not simply smaller versions of grown-ups when it comes to diagnosing and managing epilepsy. The following are important areas of difference.

• **The clinical expression of epilepsy is often atypical in infants and young children.** This is because of the incomplete development of synaptic connections, particularly between hemispheres. As a result, the adult seizure classification is not easy to apply in the very young. As the child becomes older, clinical features change, seizure type may become clearer and a child may develop additional seizure types. It may then become possible to recognize a syndrome, which will provide a clearer idea of prognosis and perhaps indicate more appropriate treatment.

• **There are certain seizure types and epilepsy syndromes which only occur or begin in childhood.** Some are rare, some serious, some benign, and some, such as childhood absence and juvenile myoclonic epilepsy, require specific treatment.

• **The diagnosis is complicated by the existence of conditions with similarities to epilepsy.** For example, approximately 2% of children experience febrile convulsions and 2% anoxic seizures. Misdiagnosis is a serious problem. Neurologists find that 10–30% of children with a diagnosis of epilepsy referred to them by other consultants do not have it. The most common causes of mistaken diagnosis are fortunately limited to a few: anoxic seizures and sleep disturbances in younger children, and syncope in teenagers.

• **The consequences of having epilepsy or a seizure are different to those in adults.** Education may be affected. Issues relating to employment or driving are not immediate, but there are implications for considering drug withdrawal before the age of eligibility to drive.

• **Adverse effects of anti-epileptic drugs may be different** and cause different problems, particularly adverse cognitive effects in relation to education.

Getting the diagnosis right

The point that diagnosis depends upon an adequate clinical history, which includes descriptions of events before, during and after the suspected seizure, has been made several times already. It is no less important in children. Obtaining a developmental history and establishing the presence or absence of possible provoking factors are particularly important, the latter especially so, since many of the conditions which cause problems in diagnosis are often responses to provocation.

Familiarity with the manifestations of basic seizure types (see Chapter 4) will make it easier to make a positive diagnosis of epilepsy (rather than 'it might be, so we'll treat it', which is what sometimes happens). It will also make a syndrome diagnosis easier. It is obviously important to be able to differentiate syndromes, but equally obvious that this requires an input of special expertise. The GP with some grasp of the 'childhood epilepsies' will be better able to recognize the need for specialist help.

Familiarity with the non-epilepsy conditions which cause problems in diagnosis is equally important (Table 7.1).

Examination and investigation

If epilepsy appears likely, examination should be directed at identifying any neurological handicap or underlying pathology if a seizure appears to be symptomatic. (Cerebral tumour is often feared, but is rare.)

In childhood, investigations are kept to a minimum.

Computed tomography and magnetic resonance imaging are difficult to carry out on small children. The latter is noisy and frightening, and general anaesthesia might be needed, so it is not undertaken lightly. They should be considered in the following:

• children with partial seizures except benign partial seizures;
• all with abnormal neurological signs;
• an electroencephalogram (EEG) with focal evidence;
• refractory seizures.

Electroencephalography is painless, fairly cheap and non-invasive. Although it cannot in many instances prove or disprove a diagnosis of epilepsy, it can frequently be a major contributor in syndrome classification, e.g. childhood absence, which has typical features of three per second spike–wave activity. A department specializing in paediatric EEGs is necessary, plus specialist interpretation to go with it.

Differential diagnosis of faints, fits and funny do's at different ages

Since differential diagnosis seems to be a serious problem and a child's age seems crucial, let us approach it this way.

Table 7.1 Non-epileptic attacks.

Temper tantrums	Benign paroxysmal vertigo
Breath-holding attacks	Night terrors
Reflex bradycardia (anoxic seizures)	Nightmares
Rocking	Sleep-walking
Head-banging	Simple faints
Tics	Hyperventilation

The first 3 months

In the first 3 months of life, it is rare to have seizures outside the neonatal period unless there is a major brain abnormality. Neonatal seizures are commonly due to metabolic derangement such as hypoglycaemia, birth asphyxia, cerebral malformation and inborn errors of metabolism. Prognosis depends on the underlying cause. GP involvement is likely to be minimal.

Three months to 4 years

From the age of 3 months to 4 years, the developing brain is extremely sensitive to environmental influences and the commonest trigger of seizures in this age group is fever.

Febrile seizures

Febrile seizures occur in 2.5% of children during the first 5 years of life [57]. There is often a family history of febrile seizures in close relatives. They are triggered by fever, are usually short-lived (less than 5 minutes), with symmetrical clonic movements, loss of consciousness and followed by rapid recovery. Usually, the fit is over by the time the child is seen by a doctor, but any seizure going on for 10 minutes or more can be dangerous. In this situation, 5–10 mg diazepam should be given rectally. Otherwise, treatment consists of cooling and paracetamol. Opinions differ about the need to admit to hospital. Certainly, it deserves consideration in a first episode because of the risk of meningitis. Thirty per cent will have a recurrence and the risk of future epilepsy is 2–5%.

A few children may suffer prolonged or asymmetrical febrile convulsions, and there is an association between these and the later development of complex partial seizures of temporal lobe origin. Children with more complex epilepsies which are difficult to treat and have a poor prognosis in terms of development may present with their first seizures triggered by fever.

Epileptic seizures

Many different types of epileptic seizure are seen in this age range, including infantile spasms (West's syndrome, Lennox–Gastaut syndrome) which are rare, myoclonic seizures, tonic and tonic–clonic seizures. It may be difficult to ascertain whether tonic–clonic seizures are secondarily generalized or primary generalized, as auras or partial seizures may not be recognized. Complex partial seizures may also be difficult to recognize at this age.

Non-epileptic attacks

Non-epileptic attacks at this age include breath-holding, reflex bradycardia, temper tantrums, rocking and head-banging.

Breath-holding attacks. In these, the child who has been hurt or thwarted will scream, hold its breath in inspiration and turn blue. If breath-holding continues, the child will become limp, lose consciousness and may twitch.

Reflex anoxic seizures. These are commonly mistaken for epilepsy and are associated with a brief period of asystole. They commonly follow an unpleasant or frightening experience. The child will suddenly become pale, 'as white as a sheet', will then fall and convulse. They may be found to have a bradycardia, and this can often be provoked in these children by pressure on the eyeball. Sometimes, other arrythmias are associated with seizures, and there may be a family history of sudden death. Electrocardiogram (ECG) abnormalities may be found.

Four to 10 years

From 4 to 10 years of age, genetic factors are important in determining the types of epilepsy presenting.

Childhood absences (petit mal) and complex partial seizures are both seen and may give rise to diagnostic difficulty. The differences have been described earlier (Chapter 4). To recap: childhood absences are almost always briefer, rarely lasting more than 30 seconds, the eyelids flutter, and although there may be automatisms in a prolonged attack, they are not as pronounced as those associated with complex partial seizures. Recovery is immediate in childhood absence and usually delayed in complex partial seizures. The EEG will usually help decide. The distinction is important, since prognosis and treatment are different.

Benign partial epilepsies are very common in this age group and are thought to account for up to 25% of all seizures presenting in this age group [48]. These are more common in boys. Seizure characteristics include unilateral paraesthesiae of tongue, lips and cheek, and unilateral clonic convulsions involving the face, lips, tongue and larynx. There is, not surprisingly, difficulty with speech. Consciousness is retained. Attacks are typically on wakening, and tonic–clonic seizures may also occur. The EEG is usually diagnostic. Treatment is effective, and patients all grow out of it by puberty.

Most generalized tonic–clonic seizures are secondarily generalized. That is, there is evidence of focal onset, although no precise lesion is defined. Usually described as 'cryptogenic', meaning 'we think we know more or less where it is coming from, but we haven't got the technology to prove it'.

The prognosis for seizures occurring in this age group is good unless associated with underlying structural abnormality.

By this age, many epilepsy syndromes will be becoming clearer and therefore careful attention should be paid to the types of seizure being experienced by an individual child.

Non-epileptic attacks now include night terrors and nightmares.

Ten years onwards and into adolescence

Over the age of 10 years, primary generalized epilepsies become more prominent, although partial epilepsies continue to be very important.

It is important to be on the lookout for juvenile myoclonic epilepsy (see Chapter 3), which requires specific treatment with sodium valproate and can be made worse by other drugs. Typical myoclonic attacks occur, involving the upper limbs, without loss of consciousness, usually on awakening or if short of sleep; 90% have tonic–clonic seizures also on awakening; 25% also have typical absence attacks.

Epilepsy with generalized tonic clonic seizures on wakening also occurs at this age. Absences persist, but true childhood absence epilepsy is less likely to present after the age of 10 years.

Non-epileptic attacks now include sleep-walking and, as we progress through the teenage years, vasovagal faints, hyperventilation and even pseudo-seizures. Faints occurring in older children are a common reason for misdiagnosis. Classical situations include: the schoolchild in morning assembly who has missed breakfast, after standing for some time, slumps to the floor with brief loss of consciousness and some twitching; or the child fainting in the toilet, remaining semi-upright and as a consequence having brief anoxic twitching.

Anti-epileptic drug treatment in childhood and adolescence

Table 7.2 shows the main anti-epileptic drug regimens in childhood. The indications and general principles are covered fully in Chapters 5

Table 7.2 Anti-epileptic drug regimens in childhood.

Drug	Starting dose	Maintenance dose	Serum levels
Sodium valproate	20 mg/kg/day in 2 divided doses	20–30 mg/kg/day in 2 or 3 divided doses	Not helpful apart from checking compliance
Carbamazepine	10 mg/kg/day in 2 divided doses	20–40 mg/kg/day in 2 or 3 divided doses	15–50 μmol/L
Ethosuximide	15 mg/kg/day in 2 divided doses	20–40 mg/kg/day in 2 or 3 divided doses	300–700 μmol/L
Clonazepam	0.02 mg/kg/day in 2 divided doses	0.1–0.2 mg/kg/day in 2 divided doses	Not helpful
Vigabatrin	40 mg/kg/day	500–2000 mg/day in 2 divided doses	Not helpful
Lamotrigine			
If on valproate	0.2 mg/kg/day for 2 weeks, then 0.5 mg/kg/day for 2 weeks	2–5 mg/kg/day	Not helpful
If on other anti-epileptic drugs	2 mg/kg/day for 2 weeks, then 5 mg/kg/day for 2 weeks	5–15 mg/kg/day	
As monotherapy	Over 12s only, see Table 5.2		
Oxcarbazepine	10 mg/kg/day 10 mg/kg weekly steps	30 mg/kg/day twice daily dosage	Value not established 50–125 μmol/L
Topiramate	0.5–1 mg/kg/day 0.5–1 mg/kg/day, fortnightly increments	Not finally defined 9–11 mg/kg/day	Value not established 6–74 μmol/L

Phenytoin, phenobarbitone, Mysoline (primidone) are not recommended for use in childhood unless under close supervision.

and 6, but there are issues in childhood and adolescence which deserve special comment.

Choosing to suit the seizure type or syndrome

Sodium valproate and carbamazepine (and phenytoin) have been shown to be equally effective against tonic–clonic seizures, whether primary or secondarily generalized, and against partial seizures. Sodium valproate is usually preferred for primary generalized epilepsy, since it is effective against childhood absence as well as tonic–clonic seizures. It is also effective against juvenile myoclonic epilepsy which carbamazepine can make worse. Vigabatrin also makes juvenile myoclonic epilepsy worse. Ethosuximide is specific for childhood absence.

The place of the newer drugs—vigabatrin, lamotrigine and gabapentin—is emerging. Vigabatrin appears useful in infantile spasms, for which it is the drug of choice, and partial epilepsy, but its neuropsychiatric side-effects are a problem as is its tendency to cause visual field defects. The Vigabatrin Paediatric Advisory Group in its latest guideline now advises sophisticated visual field assessment before prescribing vigabatrin and six monthly checks thereafter [56]. Lamotrigine has proved effective in primary generalized epilepsy including myoclonus and juvenile myoclonic epilepsy. Gabapentin's role is less certain; although it has fewer side-effects, its efficacy is modest. It is useful as add-on treatment for partial seizures, but is ineffective in most generalized seizures and in myoclonus.

More recently, topiramate has been shown to be very effective over a wide spectrum of anti-epileptic activity, both in partial and generalized epilepsy —including typical absence and myoclonus. It is effective in children, including the Lennox–Gastaut syndrome; although there can be problems with side-effects, these appear to be less of a problem in children. Oxcarbazepine, now available in the UK, has the same range of effectiveness as carbamazepine but with less severe side-effects and fewer interactions.

Choosing to suit the individual

Although attaining seizure control is the fundamental aim, avoiding drug side-effects, particularly those causing sedation or dulling intellect, comes a close second. There is little to choose between sodium valproate and carbamazepine, which are tolerated reasonably well. Because of sedative effects, phenytoin and phenobarbitone should now only be used as a last resort. Other side-effects of phenytoin, especially cosmetic, reduce its usefulness. Of the newer drugs, vigabatrin can cause behavioural disturbance, but lamotrigine and gabapentin are well tolerated.

Sodium valproate can have endocrine effects, with alterations in sex hormone levels resulting in anovulatory cycles, amenorrhoea, polycystic ovary syndrome, and it may lead to weight gain. Adolescence is generally associated with sexual activity, and the effects of enzyme-inducing drugs on oral contraception need to be anticipated, as well as the potential effects of drugs in pregnancy.

Ease of use

It is important to avoid the need for medication to be taken during the day at school or college. It causes practical difficulties and leads to poor compliance. Standard preparations of sodium valproate and carbamazepine can be effective in a twice-daily regime, but the sustained-release preparations are probably better, and in any case may produce fewer sedative side-effects.

Coming off medication

Withdrawal of medication can be attempted in most children who have been seizure-free for 2 years (at 2 years after stopping, 75% will be seizure-free). Juvenile myoclonic epilepsy is an exception and relapse is likely, so treatment is best continued.

Living with epilepsy in childhood

The immediate impact on parents of a diagnosis of epilepsy in a child can be devastating: fears that the child might die during a seizure, might suffer brain damage, might have a brain tumour, might become mentally disabled; fear, shame, guilt; worries about the stigma, of being 'different'. Later, other practical concerns and questions arise, to do with living with the diagnosis and its consequences. Chapter 8 offers a checklist approach to covering these issues, and Chapter 9 provides answers to many of the questions commonly asked. The following are important immediate concerns.

Initial concerns

The starting point must be to convey to the family that the majority of children who develop epilepsy are otherwise normal and should be able to lead reasonably normal lives. Also, that many grow out of it. At this stage, immediate advice must be given about such things as what to do if the child has a fit, sensible avoidance of danger and the consideration of referral to a patient organization and epilepsy nurse specialist (if you are lucky enough to have one). Continuity of support for the psychological and social problems are as important as getting the treatment right.

Overprotection is understandable and is common, especially in children whose seizures are not controlled. The vulnerable child may withdraw and avoid competition, while the overprotected may become angry and manipulative. Dependency has to be resisted. It is not uncommon to see adults who have had epilepsy since childhood attending a clinic escorted by ageing parents who do all the talking (Fig. 7.1).

Other brothers or sisters must not be ignored in the concern for the child with epilepsy; their attitudes and fears need attention. Not infrequently, siblings may have an unrecognized anxiety that a brother or sister might die during a fit, particularly if they have had to cope alone when a seizure has occurred. (Useful booklets and videos are available to assist in teaching other children about epilepsy and how they can help.) The role of schools and teachers is important in helping a child to grow to independence, and parents need to discuss their child's needs with teachers. School nurses and

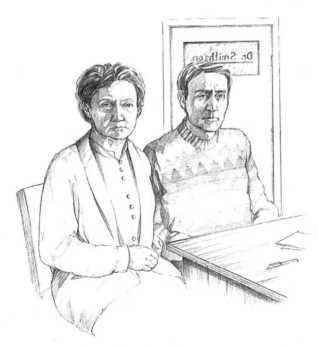

Fig. 7.1 Many parents of people with epilepsy are overprotective, and it is not uncommon for an adult patient to be escorted to the surgery by an elderly parent.

epilepsy specialist nurses can be useful allies in this. It can be an enormous help if teachers can recognize absence attacks or complex partial seizures, and ensure that a child catches up on what has been missed.

Adolescence

Adolescence can be a difficult enough time without the added complication of epilepsy. Often, a teenager with previous epilepsy will still be treated as if younger. The onset of epilepsy may coincide with puberty, when the youngster striving for independence finds parents responding with overprotection. Anxiety, loss of dignity, being made to feel different and low esteem will all feature. Anger, resentment and denial are common, and as a consequence medication may not be taken regularly, sometimes as part of a battle against parental authority.

Clearly, advice, information and support are needed in abundance, but adolescence is 'rebellion time', and advice may be unwelcome. Besides, who gives it? Even if a paediatrician or paediatric neurologist had previously provided good support, they may no longer be involved. There are good arguments for careful 'handover' arrangements between child services and adults, as are offered by the adolescent epilepsy service in Liverpool, but in the absence of such a service, dealing with adolescents with epilepsy can be a considerable challenge for the GP, or perhaps the practice nurse.

It is hoped that most adolescents will achieve insight and acceptance, but emotional and practical problems will remain. Independence has its attendant risks—taking holidays without parents and going away to college. Leaving home is even more stressful than for other young people—being different, taking medication, 'What do I tell my new friends?', 'What if I have a fit in front of them all?'

Epilepsy in women

Epilepsy in women deserves particular attention because of the effects of epilepsy and anti-epileptic drugs on fertility, contraception and pregnancy, and also because of variation in seizure activity in relationship to the menstrual cycle in a few women. In addition, there is the greater risk of osteoporosis, the role of HRT and its safety.

The particular problems associated with epilepsy in women have attracted increasing attention in recent years and are fully reviewed in the latest guidelines from the Women with Epilepsy Guidelines Development Group [58].

Epilepsy, the menstrual cycle and fertility

Both epilepsy and its treatment can alter the menstrual cycle and affect fertility. Fertility rates are lower in women with epilepsy than in the general population, and there is a higher incidence of anovulatory cycles in women with partial seizures of temporal lobe origin. The prevalence of polycystic ovary syndrome may be higher in women with epilepsy, and particularly in those taking sodium valproate (especially if taken before the age of 20).

Catamenial epilepsy

There is little doubt that some women with epilepsy have more seizures just before or during menstruation; indeed, a few only appear to experience seizures at this time. No one seems to be certain why, and some experts doubt the relationship. In practical terms, if substantial doses of first-line anti-epileptic drugs fail to control such seizures, then clobazam often works in a divided dose of 20–30 mg/day started 3 or 4 days before the anticipated onset of seizures and continued for 7 days. Also useful is acetazolamide 250 mg three times daily starting 8–10 days before the period is expected and continued for 10 days.

Sexuality

Although sexual desire and sexual arousal may be affected by epilepsy or its treatment, the majority of women with epilepsy have normal sex lives.

Contraception

There is no reason why women with epilepsy taking anti-epileptic medication should not take oral contraceptives. A problem arises with those drugs which induce liver enzyme activity and increase the metabolism of oestrogens and progestogens, rendering the combined pill or progestogen-only pill unreliable. Carbamazepine, phenytoin, the barbiturates (this includes primidone), oxcarbazepine and topiramate fall into this category, but sodium valproate, benzodiazepines, vigabatrin, gabapentin, lamotrigine, and tiagabine do not. The answer is for patients taking carbamazepine, phenytoin or barbiturates to take a higher dosage of oestrogen and progestogen as follows.

The combined contraceptive pill and enzyme-inducing anti-epileptic drugs

A dose of at least 50 µg of oestrogen should be given. If breakthrough bleeding occurs, the dose should be increased. In the first instance, a 'tricycle regimen' can be tried, i.e. three packets without a break. If necessary, up to 100 µg of oestrogen can be given. However, even a regular menstrual cycle is not an entirely reliable guide to effective contraception, and if absolute certainty is required, blood progesterone levels on day 21 of the cycle are said to give the answer. Guidance on appropriate levels must be sought from the local laboratory.

The progestogen-only pill and injections

When given together with liver enzyme-inducing drugs, the simplest thing to do is double the dose of the progestogen-only pill. Depot progestogen should be given every 10 weeks instead every 12 weeks. Norplant is not approved in these circumstances. If appropriate, the morning-after pill can be used, but in a slightly higher dose if enzyme-inducing anti-epileptic drugs are being taken.

Epilepsy and pregnancy

Most women with epilepsy can expect a normal pregnancy, without any increase in seizures, and have a healthy child [59]. However, there is a slightly increased risk of complications and malformations. The incidence of malformations in the general population is less than 3%. The risk of the latter is increased by anti-epileptic drugs, particularly when several are being taken at the same time. Infants of mothers on anti-epileptic drugs have at least double the chance of being born with a malformation; fortunately, the majority of malformations are minor.

Ideally, a woman with epilepsy considering becoming pregnant should be referred for specialist advice, or at least receive full information and counselling. Careful management of pregnancy is desirable both from the obstetric and the epilepsy points of view.

Preconceptual counselling

Preconceptual counselling is not something that we are very good at. Usually, we realize it would have been a good idea when the patient presents already pregnant, which is a bit late for choices, and the anti-epileptic drugs will have done whatever they were going to do. Now that the relative risks both for pregnancy and the effects of drugs are better understood, it has become important to provide information and advice in time. It is worth noting that litigation has been undertaken because of failure to warn about the possibility of anti-epileptic drugs causing malformations in infants.

When choosing anti-epileptic medication for a woman of childbearing age, the consequences for future pregnancies should be borne in mind. **A reminder should be given to seek advice about medication before considering pregnancy, and it might just be wise to record the giving of the advice in the records.** GPs might consider advising women and girls at risk when reviewing their repeat prescriptions.

When seen prior to pregnancy, the need for continuing medication should be considered. Any changes in anti-epileptic drugs should be completed before conception. Expert advice is desirable before considering withdrawal. If, as is likely, the decision is to continue medication, the patient is best on the smallest effective dose of a single anti-epileptic drug, certainly in the first few months of pregnancy (Fig. 7.2).

All of the major anti-epileptic drugs—carbamazepine, valproate, phenytoin and phenobarbitone—are teratogenic, but the risks are greater with poly-therapy [59]. Phenytoin and phenobarbitone are liable to cause heart defects

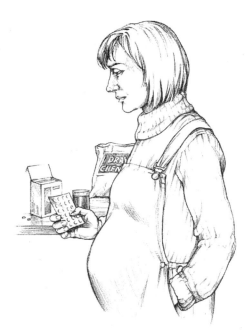

Fig. 7.2 Medication and pregnancy.

and cleft palate (1–2%). There is a slightly increased risk of spina bifida in patients on sodium valproate (1–1.5%) and carbamazepine (1%), and patients on these two drugs should take folic acid before any pregnancy and for the first 12 weeks, in a dose of 4–5 mg/day. Women on sodium valproate and carbamazepine should be counselled and told that they will be offered antenatal screening (α-fetoprotein and ultrasound scanning) during pregnancy. It is not known whether vigabatrin, gabapentin, lamotrigine, topiramate, oxcarbazepine or levetiracetam are associated with a risk of foetal abnormality.

During pregnancy

It is important that there is a co-ordinated approach to the management of pregnancy and labour. The epilepsy specialist nurse, where available, should be responsible for liaison between clinicians, midwives, and later health visitors.

In most women, there will be no worsening of seizure control during pregnancy. One-third will have an increase in seizures, but this may be due to medication being left off purposefully in order to protect the baby, or alternatively because of loss of sleep, or morning sickness preventing the retention of a morning dose. In others, there is no obvious explanation, but it tends to be associated with low anti-epileptic drug levels early in pregnancy.

As far as anti-epileptic treatment is concerned, once pregnancy is established, it is unwise to make radical changes, but to adjust the dose of existing medication according to need. Anti-epileptic drug serum levels fall in pregnancy for a number of reasons: increased liver metabolism, increase in blood volume, reduction of albumin concentration causing reduced protein binding and, of course, non-compliance. But it is nevertheless more sensible to adjust dosage according to clinical need, i.e. to increase it if seizures increase, rather than to treat according to serum levels. If, however, a women is seizure-free and a single seizure would jeopardize keeping a driver's licence, there is good reason to maintain serum levels within the therapeutic range rather than to increase dosage in response to seizures. After delivery, the dose should be reduced to the pre-pregnancy level unless there has been improved control on the new dose.

Because of the risk of haemorrhagic disease of the newborn in the offspring of women on enzyme-inducing drugs, a dose of 20 mg per day of Vit K1 should be given orally in the last month of pregnancy. Infants born of women with epilepsy should receive 1 mg Vit K1 intramuscularly at birth.

Fits and the foetus

The foetus appears to be relatively resistant to the effects of maternal seizures, although there is a risk from falls.

During labour

A slightly increased risk of seizures during labour is associated with failure to take medication, poor absorption of drugs, lack of sleep and dehydration. For these reasons, it is better for childbirth to take place in hospital. Having said that, there is much to be said for the father-to-be, if he is in attendance as is nowadays customary, to take responsibility for reminding hospital staff that it is time for his partner's tablets.

Baby care

Breast-feeding is safe for the baby, since breast milk contains anti-epileptic drugs only in small concentrations, less than the intra-uterine dose. Phenobarbitone can be a problem, and if the baby is excessively drowsy alternate breast and bottle feeds are helpful. Where active epilepsy is a problem, bottle-feeding may have a place. If, for example, lack of sleep triggers seizures, the partner can share the task of feeding the baby. Coping with babies and small children, as well as having seizures, presents special problems. There may be a risk of dropping the baby during a seizure, and it may be better to feed a baby while sitting on the floor. It is also better to wash and change the baby on the floor, and only bath the baby when someone else is around. Ideally, these issues should all be discussed before the baby is born.

Epilepsy and the menopause

The effects of epilepsy on the menopause and the effects of hormonal changes on epilepsy cannot be reliably predicted. Some women find the menopause has no effect on seizure frequency, others that there is an increase or a recurrence, or even a remission. Women with epilepsy are at risk of bone demineralization, especially if they are taking enzyme-inducing anti-epileptic drugs. It is suggested that all post-menopausal women with epilepsy should receive HRT (combined oestrogen and progestogen) if it is clinically indicated.

Epilepsy and learning disability

Since the emptying of the large mental handicap hospitals most people with learning disability in the UK are now in the community and should be on the list of a general practitioner. Actually, even before this, the majority were already supported by their families in the community. An average GP will now have six or seven patients with moderate, severe and profound learning disabilities [60]; about 25% of these will also have epilepsy [61]. A group practice of four doctors will therefore have six or seven patients who have both epilepsy and learning disability. As if that were not enough, they are likely to have more than their share of general health problems, sensory impairments, mental health problems (including challenging behaviour), cerebral palsy and other physical disabilities.

The fundamental problem in managing patients with learning disability is in communication. In a large proportion of these patients communication has to be through a third person—a family or professional carer. Kerr, in his useful review on managing epilepsy in patients with learning disability, describes it as 'management by proxy' [62]. **The information needed to establish a diagnosis, recognize the effectiveness of treatment or drug side-effects is through observing behaviour** rather than speech.

The epilepsy

The classification of epilepsy syndromes is not so useful in this group. The epilepsy tends to be severe, with frequent attacks, and is refractory in 75% despite drug treatment [61]. There is a broad range of seizure types, with a high prevalence of generalized epilepsy, including tonic–clonic and the more difficult atonic/tonic generalized seizures. Many experience more than one type of seizure.

Anti-epileptic drugs and learning disability

There is general agreement to avoid phenobarbitone and concern about vigabatrin and its potential for behavioural side-effects. Patients on vigabatrin are now advised to have six-monthly checks of peripheral vision because of the very high risk of visual loss (see Chapter 6, pages 76–77). This hardly seems a practical proposition for many in this group. The choice of drug should be suited to the needs of the individual (see Chapter 5, page 52), and preferably as monotherapy. Obesity is a common problem in learning disability and valproate may make this worse, especially in young women. Valproate is also associated with the polycystic ovary syndrome (see Chapter 6, page 71), and the issues of contraception and pregnancy should not be overlooked (see above, Epilepsy in women). There is much to be said for using a drug with a wide spectrum of action if the seizure type is unknown. Some of the newer drugs with fewer side-effects may prove helpful for these patients in the future. Many patients (and their carers) find blood tests very upsetting, and generally blood level monitoring should be avoided if it is possible, but since many are unable to talk about side-effects and become toxic on small increases of drugs (notably phenytoin), blood tests have an important place, especially when titrating the dose or adding a new drug.

Behaviour, seizures and side-effects

Disentangling behaviour caused by a seizure from that caused by medication, and from behaviour which is unrelated to either, is not easy. An individual exhibiting complex behaviour, for example, undressing inappropriately or fidgeting, might be thought to be having a complex partial seizure. But in this population it could be seen as an aspect of normal behaviour. The possibility that drugs might cause behavioural problems is of particular concern, but behavioural changes are very common in these individuals anyway. Distinguishing between drug-induced and normal changes in behaviour is very difficult but important, since it might lead to withdrawing drugs unnecessarily.

Common health problems and physical difficulties which affect behaviour and epilepsy

- Feeding and swallowing difficulties can lead to compliance problems for both epilepsy and other medication (including mental health treatment).
- Nutritional problems and constipation can affect behaviour and the latter often seems to make epilepsy worse.
- Infections of the urinary tract and upper respiratory tract are often insidious, worsening behaviour and epilepsy.
- Difficulties with co-ordination and mobility may be exacerbated by anti-epileptic medication.

Taking a detailed history from the family and carers is really important (see Appendix 4), as you need to know what the 'normal' baseline behaviour pattern is for the individual before you and the carers can make sense of any apparent change. A learning disability nurse can be of invaluable help in this (see Chapter 11). Generally, it is better to wait until an issue is clear before acting. Sudden changes in drug therapy can lead to an exacerbation of seizures and/or side-effects. Carers can be helped if they know what to expect, and if they do, the information they feed back will be more useful. For example, if vigabatrin is prescribed they can be warned to watch for unusual behaviour. If lamotrigine is given with carbamazepine they should be warned about the confusion that might be caused by double vision.

Kerr and Todd [63] suggest the following three areas of questioning when faced with someone with learning disability, epilepsy and challenging behaviour.

1 *Is it behaviour caused by seizures?*

Does it happen just before or after seizures?

Can you rule out any other obvious cause, e.g. somebody has upset them?

Does the person look drowsy or confused when the behaviour occurs/ before/after?

Does the person sleep afterwards?

Is the behaviour the same each time?

2 *Is it behaviour caused by medication?*

When did the problem start, i.e. did it coincide with changes in medication?

What is the individual like in between episodes of problem behaviour—too drowsy, too active?

Is the individual off food/sleep?

Does the behaviour occur after taking the medication?

3 *Behaviour independent of seizures/medication?*

Is it a long-standing problem?

Do changes in medication or numbers of seizures appear to have no effect on the behaviour?

A seizure/behaviour diary kept by carers based upon the above has been found to be a useful tool in understanding what is going on.

What are we trying to accomplish?

The basic aim is to achieve a balance between controlling seizures and freedom from drug side-effects for the benefit of both the individual and those living with and caring for him or her. Seizure control is not everything—the occasional partial seizure is relatively unimportant compared with the side-effects of medication. Carers worry that drugs might worsen learning skills, or that treatment to reduce seizures will put the patient to sleep. The effects of drugs on learning skills tend to be of greater concern in managing the more able patients, whereas getting control of seizures without putting them to sleep is more important for the more severely disabled.

Carers worry about and desire information about the link between disturbed behaviour and epilepsy and therefore need support and information. This education and support is very important, and although those in group homes, it is hoped, get this from a 'named nurse', support for those in the community is patchy. Community learning disability nurses undertake this role with people referred to them, but many struggle on without help. Support groups for families of people with learning disability are available here and there, and are often more helpful than epilepsy support groups, who are not always as welcoming of people with learning disability. Learning disability epilepsy specialist nurses (see Chapter 11), working closely with specialist epilepsy services, have an increasing role in co-ordinating care for local populations with learning disability who also have epilepsy.

What can the non-specialist do?

This all sounds as if it should be a job led by specialists in both learning disability and epilepsy. Ordinary doctors, including GPs, are sure to feel out of their depth. As in other aspects of epilepsy care, non-specialists can contribute best within an overall structure which includes specialist services. Locally agreed guidelines for epilepsy management, specialist epilepsy nurses, learning disability nurses with epilepsy training and community learning disability epilepsy specialist nurses are desirable. GPs should consider pressing for these services through primary care groups (PCGs), and encourage referral of isolated patients and families to the learning disability services and support groups.

Whatever is available, there are practical contributions to be made:

• Information and education about epilepsy and drug effects are vital for the carers. The disability team, specialist nurses and practice nurses may provide this, and material can be obtained from the epilepsy associations.

• Being available and supportive—having a person who is easy to contact in the practice, such as the practice nurse.

• Being prepared to review patients from time to time to identify problems.

• Looking at compliance and how drugs are taken. Many patients have problems eating and are difficult to persuade to take tablets; often drugs can be taken less frequently, perhaps in a long-acting preparation, with benefit.

• If there is no specialist involved, seizures are uncontrolled and a drug with few side-effects is being prescribed in sub-optimal dosage, consider increasing it in small steps.

• Question recommendations to make sudden drug changes, particularly if from a non-epilepsy specialist source such as an A&E department.

• Be prepared to question the suggested use of very sedative drugs or drugs with bad side-effects.

• Show that you value these patients particularly.

Epilepsy in the elderly

Epilepsy in old age is as important as at any other time of life, and is associated with its own particular problems, which often go unrecognized and deserve attention. Contrary to popular belief, epilepsy is not only common in old age, but its prevalence actually increases with age. There is a steeper rise in incidence from the age of 50 years onwards, and the National General Practice Study of Epilepsy found that almost one-quarter of newly diagnosed epilepsy was in those over 60 years of age [27]. Of an individual GP's 10–15 patients with epilepsy, two or three will be over 65 years, and there will be about one new case in the elderly every 2–4 years.

Diagnosis

Diagnosis can be difficult in the elderly. For one thing, the history may be inadequate, especially in the absence of a witnessed account, for example, when an old person lives alone. Cardiovascular causes of episodic loss of consciousness are more common in old age, and distinguishing these from seizures can be difficult. The usual distinctions between faints and fits do not always apply. Simple faints typically have a slow onset, contrasting with the sudden onset of most seizures, but cardiac syncope can be quite abrupt.

Causes of epilepsy in the elderly

Cerebrovascular disease is the most common cause of epilepsy in the elderly [27,64,65]. It accounts for about 30–50% of cases overall, and nearly three-quarters of cases in which a definite cause can be found. A seizure may be the first manifestation of otherwise silent cerebrovascular disease, and an otherwise unexplained seizure may warn of future stroke. Therefore, any elderly patient with unexplained seizures should be screened for cerebrovascular risk factors, and consideration given to providing long-term treatment with aspirin. Stroke alone leads to early seizures in 4% of patients and 10% of stroke cases have seizures within 5 years [65].

Cerebral tumours are a more common cause of epilepsy than in the young, and are associated with seizures in between 5 and 15% of cases of newly diagnosed epilepsy in the elderly [27,65]. Most, but not all, of these are metastatic.

Other important causes of seizures in old age include toxic and metabolic causes (of these, alcohol is important at any age), pyrexia and pneumonia (with hypoxia); many drugs may cause confusion and convulsions.

Features of seizures in old age

At least three-quarters of seizures in the elderly are symptomatic, and are due to focal underlying cerebral lesions [27], most of which are cerebrovascular in origin. Classifications of seizures and syndromes, important though they are in childhood and early adult life in indicating prognosis and determining treatment, have little practical relevance in old age.

The effects of seizures may be more pronounced. Post-ictal states are often prolonged beyond the traditional 24 hours (sometimes as long as a week) and Todd's phenomena are more common, especially post-ictal hemiparesis.

Consequences of seizures in old age

Seizures are more likely to lead to injury from falling; old bones can be brittle. Since the elderly often live alone, consideration may need to be given to devising means of summoning help. Providing supervision without reducing independence is important. The impact of developing epilepsy may be seen as a portent of inevitable decline, and the fear of having further seizures may lead to loss of confidence and independence.

The elderly may be more likely to feel stigmatized by the diagnosis and associate epilepsy with mental problems. This, too, can lead to withdrawal and self-imposed isolation. Overprotective attitudes of friends, relatives and carers may add to this, and may lead to decreased activity. There is a danger of less involvement in rearing grandchildren and increased susceptibility to interference in personal affairs.

Elderly people may be particularly dependent upon the motor car, and so, if the individual developing epilepsy is the only licence-holder, two people may become housebound.

Management

A positive approach is important and totally justified in most cases because the prognosis for control is usually good. It is essential to provide adequate information and be at pains to anticipate and correct misunderstandings which the elderly often have about the nature and consequences of having epilepsy. The section on counselling (Chapter 8) provides more information, but the following list is helpful.
- The nature of seizures should be explained.
- Provide reassurance that, in the majority of cases, seizures do not indicate serious brain damage, psychiatric disease or dementia.

• Explain that seizures can almost always be controlled by medication.

• Advice should be given to avoid situations which might precipitate seizures, such as inadequate sleep or excess alcohol. It is worth pointing out that although alcohol might increase the side-effects of medication, the latter should never be left off simply because alcohol has been taken. Moderation is best.

• A patient who drives a motor car must be advised to inform the Driving and Vehicle Licensing Agency (DVLA), and given advice about the current regulations (see Chapter 8, page 116, for details of driving regulations).

• Anticipate and attempt to counter possible loss of confidence and voluntary restriction of activity. Advise avoidance *only* of those activities which would lead to danger if a seizure occurred.

• Relatives, neighbours and carers should be taught how to deal with seizures.

• Foster an interdisciplinary approach. Involve liaison nurses, social workers and occupational therapists, to review home circumstances and needs, e.g. in assessing for potential sources of danger.

• Supply contact information about the British Epilepsy Association or other epilepsy organizations and any local support groups.

Medication

Since the population of elderly with epilepsy will include those diagnosed in early life as well as recently, a GP may have patients on a wide range of anti-epileptic drugs, some of which would no longer be used by choice. These, unless proving harmful, are best left alone, but the possible interaction with other drugs should be borne in mind.

For newly diagnosed patients, it is desirable to choose an anti-epileptic drug which will be effective for the particular seizure type, have the minimum of cognitive side-effects, be easy to take, not cause disaster if occasionally forgotten and not interact with other medication. Since most newly diagnosed epilepsy in old age is localization-related, any first-line anti-epileptic drug will be suitable. Carbamazepine and sodium valproate are the best alternatives among established drugs. Of the two, carbamazepine has some disadvantages as an enzyme inducer and may interact with other medication. It also occasionally causes hyponatraemia, and is therefore not desirable in heart failure. Phenytoin, although used less in general, is popular with many geriatricians who consider it to be quite well tolerated by the elderly. It has, of course, the advantage of a once-daily dosage, but like carbamazepine may have interactions. Of the newer drugs, both lamotrigine and gabapentin are likely to prove useful in the elderly. Lamotrigine is now licensed for monotherapy but not yet specifically for the elderly, and gabapentin is remarkably free from side-effects, but not yet licensed for monotherapy at all. The tendency of vigabatrin to cause behavioural problems in a proportion of patients does not recommend its use in the elderly.

8 Living with Epilepsy: Information, Support and Counselling

Epilepsy carries unique burdens for patients and their families. Apart from having to put up with seizures, many feel stigmatized. A small number have other disabilities, such as learning disability associated with the underlying neurological disturbance responsible for the epilepsy. Others face problems in education, employment and in everyday life.

The need for information and counselling

The extensive evidence about what patients lack or feel that they want has been fully explored earlier (Chapter 1). In summary, patients and families expressed the need for more information and more services; information about epilepsy and its treatment and information to help them cope. They wanted closer follow-up and support when changing medication, and someone other than a doctor to talk to, such as a specialist nurse.

The value of information and support

The experience of the community-based specialist epilepsy nursing service in Doncaster is that 'being helped to understand and to cope with having epilepsy is as important to patients and families as improving seizure control'. Common reactions from those using this service included: 'Why couldn't someone have told me this 20 years ago!' and 'This is the first time anyone has explained anything'. The effects of this sort of service are more than the provision of 'tender loving care', although the knowledge that 'there is somebody there, who can be contacted' appears to be greatly appreciated. Accurate information removes a great deal of fear and anxiety, and reduced stress reduces seizures. Understanding how drugs work, and how to remember to take them, improves compliance and seizure control. Pointing out what may trigger an individual's seizures, e.g. tiredness and lack of sleep, may seem obvious, but has often not been considered. Assistance in completing applications for benefits or services can make the difference between getting them or not.

Although this is all, admittedly, desirable, who has the time when there are 12–15 existing patients per GP and one or two new patients a year? Say half an hour or more each, perhaps more than once. You might agree that the practice nurse might take some of it on, but then he or she is busy as well, and might need training. This is all true of course, but perhaps you might consider making a start? At least provide information about the epilepsy associations, and perhaps lobby the health authority or board to provide epilepsy services which include specialist nurses or counsellors (see Chapter 10).

What information and support? How to supply it

Difficulty in providing adequate information to patients is not unique to epilepsy, but no one can doubt that it has particular problems. For a start, there is a great deal to convey, both about epilepsy and its consequences, and much of it is complicated.

Only so much information can be taken in on one occasion, and little may be absorbed when the patient and relatives are having to take in the impact of the diagnosis of epilepsy. For patients and families, the questions at the forefront are likely to include: 'Will he or she die in one of these attacks?', 'Is it a tumour on the brain or a haemorrhage?', 'Will it lead to mental illness?', 'What about my job?' The doctor's explanations and instructions may not be remembered.

Later, when the immediate impact has been absorbed, patients and relatives may not be sure what questions to ask, they may feel lost, uncertain of the consequences of having epilepsy, and unaware of sources of help.

The implications of having epilepsy are different not only for individuals, but also for the same individual at different times of life: the child at school, the adult dependent upon the motor car for a job. The difficulties facing a 15-year-old schoolgirl who is a keen swimmer will change after a few years, when she begins to consider such things as oral contraception, marriage and having children of her own.

The remainder of this chapter outlines common and important needs for information and help for those with epilepsy, their families and carers. It offers a checklist approach to providing and exploring the need for information, and complements Chapter 9, which provides answers to common questions.

A checklist approach

A checklist approach is essential to ensure that important basic information is not overlooked, either at the time of diagnosis or as life and circumstances change. **One of the most important items on the checklist is referral to an appropriate epilepsy association.** The epilepsy associations are an important source of information and material for health professionals as well as patients, offering literature searches, leaflets, videos and professional membership (see 'Sources of Help and Advice', Appendix 1).

Table 8.1 shows the checklist used in Doncaster, and Fig. 8.1 a useful alternative list supplied to GPs by the Epilepsy Association of Scotland. The following discussion is structured around Table 8.1.

About epilepsy

What epilepsy is

Patients and relatives are often given no explanation, however simple, about what may have caused the epilepsy or what epilepsy is. It is important to make sure that the patient, or parents, understand very definitely that the patient has epilepsy if that is the case. Single seizures require explanation and attention, but epilepsy is generally defined as a tendency to recurring seizures. It often helps to put this into perspective by mentioning that about 5% of us will experience a seizure at some time in our lives. As to cause, if this is known (e.g. a focus of damage from a head injury or stroke), this

Table 8.1 Information checklist.

About epilepsy	*Lifestyle implications*
What epilepsy is	Employment
What happens in a seizure	Education
First aid in a seizure	Safety—home/outdoors/school/work
When to get medical help	Driving
Prognosis	Sport
	The pill/contraception
Precipitating factors	Pregnancy
Stress	Inheritance
Lack of sleep	Sexuality
Boredom	
Alcohol	*About drugs*
Missing tablets	How they work
Menstruation	Importance of compliance
Photosensitivity (television flicker)	Side-effects
Missed meals (hypoglycaemia)	Free prescriptions

Sources of help: literature from drug companies; epilepsy associations (see Appendix 1); support groups.

Epilepsy Association of Scotland

EPILEPSY CHECKLIST

This checklist aims to assist GP's, other doctors and community teams in meeting the information needs of epilepsy patients and their carers.

THE DIAGNOSIS   Does the patient/carer understand ....
- ★ that the diagnosis is epilepsy?
- ★ what epilepsy is?
- ★ what their own seizures are like?
- ★ what their own seizures are called?

THE MEDICATION   Does the patient/carer know ....
- ★ the purpose of the medication?
- ★ the importance of compliance?
- ★ about possible drug side effects?
- ★ about drug interactions (eg antiepileptic medication and oral contraceptives)?
- ★ what to do if
            - a dose is missed?
            - vomiting occurs?
            - a trip abroad is planned?
- ★ that the medication is free?

BASIC INFORMATION   Has the patient/carer had ....
- ★ a basic information booklet?
- ★ a chance to see an epilepsy video?
- ★ first aid instruction/demonstration?
- ★ information on legal restrictions for driving and certain jobs?

LIFE-STYLE   Has guidance been given on ......
- ★ leading a full and active life?
- ★ adopting a moderate approach to alcohol?
- ★ having regular and sufficient sleep?
- ★ safety in the home (consider for each individual fires/radiators, bathing/showering, stairs, pillows, cookers, locked doors etc)?
- ★ safety/risk for sport and recreation (consider for each individual swimming, cycling, riding etc)?
- ★ implications of epilepsy (eg for relationships and parenthood)?

ONGOING DIALOGUE   Has the patient/carer been encouraged to ....
- ★ return with questions?
- ★ keep a record of seizures?
- ★ report changes in seizure pattern and general health to GP?

FURTHER HELP   Is the patient/carer aware ....
- ★ that additional support and information on all the above topics can be obtained from:

THE EPILEPSY ASSOCIATION OF SCOTLAND
NATIONAL HEADQUARTERS
48 GOVAN ROAD, GLASGOW G51 1JL, TEL 041 427 4911

Fig. 8.1 Epilepsy Association of Scotland checklist.

is straightforward and easy to explain. Some of the childhood epilepsies may be genetically determined. For most, the underlying cause will not be known, although a focus of damage or disturbance in the brain may be implied from the seizure type. (Causes are referred to in Chapter 2.)

What happens during a seizure

The patient may have never seen a seizure and may be bewildered at the impact it has on others. It is useful to use an analogy such as electrical activity affecting certain parts of the brain. It is a particularly useful way of explaining the symptoms experienced during a spread of seizure activity from a localized epileptic focus to the rest of the brain. Figures 3.1, 3.2 and 3.4 may be found useful in explaining what happens. A good example would be a partial seizure such as an aura, starting in the temporal lobe, evolving to a tonic–clonic seizure. Of course, the patient will be mainly interested in what happens in one of his or her own seizures, and if a focus is apparent from the seizure type or tests, it may be possible to describe what happens in a way relevant to the patient.

First aid and what to do

Relatives and friends need to know how to cope with seizures, sometimes of different types, and when to get medical help. The anxieties and fears of children in a family when a parent or sibling has a seizure are often overlooked. It is important that they have a share in explanations and are reassured that the one they love is not going to die, and especially when they are alone with them.

There are more don'ts than dos, and these need to be made clear.

During a tonic–clonic seizure, onlookers should NOT:
• move the patient unless he or she is in danger of further injury, e.g. from fire or traffic;
• lift the patient or try to restrict movement;
• place anything in the mouth or give anything by mouth.

During a tonic–clonic seizure onlookers should:
• leave clear space around the patient;
• put something under the head and neck to give support;
• turn the patient on one side in order to assist breathing and aid general recovery once the seizure has taken its course; wipe away any mucus;
• time the seizure.

An ambulance or medical help is not usually necessary unless the patient does not regain consciousness or the seizure continues for more than 10 minutes, or the patient goes into further seizures.

On recovery, the patient should be told what has happened, be reassured and allowed to rest if necessary. Some people are very quickly able to carry on with normal activities, others need a longer period to recover.

Absence seizures and complex partial seizures do not usually require any action other than staying with the individual until recovery. If during or after a complex partial seizure there is a prolonged period of altered consciousness and automatic behaviour, the person should be accompanied and if it is necessary, gently led away from any danger.

Prognosis

What will or may happen in the future is vitally important to anyone with epilepsy. It is, however, difficult to predict, especially at the outset, and everyone is different. (Prognosis is fully discussed in Chapter 2.) **In general, the prospect for most people is encouraging, both for seizure control and even for remission.** The prognosis for seizure control in new patients is 70–86% and about 60–70% of patients will enter remission. Factors influencing prognosis include age of onset, seizure and syndrome type. Onset in the first five years of life tends to have a poor prognosis; otherwise, childhood epilepsy is more likely to remit than epilepsy starting in adult life. Remission rates of 60–80% have been shown for tonic–clonic seizures alone, compared with only 20–60% for complex partial seizures; 70–80% of childhood absence epilepsy will remit. Not surprisingly, epilepsy associated with other neurological handicap is less likely to remit.

Precipitating factors

The commonest precipitants of seizures are stress, boredom, alcohol, missed tablets, lack of sleep, menstruation and hypoglycaemia from missed meals. Patients need to be aware of these factors and attempt to adjust their lifestyle.

Stress is common in epilepsy. Newly diagnosed patients find it difficult to come to terms with their condition, while chronic patients face more difficulties than the rest of us. Keeping busy reduces seizures as long as overtiredness is avoided.

People with epilepsy need regular sleep and so it is inadvisable for some to work shifts. A combination of late nights, alcohol and missed tablets can be a recipe for disaster. Often, tablets are missed before a party because the label on the bottle says 'Not to be taken with alcohol'. **Tablets should never be missed**, and for most patients a few drinks in moderation are not a problem.

Seizures can be triggered by flickering lights or television in some individuals (photosensitive epilepsy). This can be avoided by sitting at least 3 metres away from the set, covering one eye to adjust the set, using a remote control and placing a table lamp on or behind the set. Outdoors, polarized sunglasses (not ordinary tinted) may be of help. Small television screens are safer and antiglare computer screens can protect. It is advisable not to use a computer for more than 30–40 minutes without a break.

Lifestyle implications

Many families become overprotective of the sufferer and some people fail to become independent, particularly if epilepsy has started in childhood. This affects all aspects of life—education, leisure, making outside relationships and employment. If adequate information is given to both family and patient, the patient can and should be encouraged to lead as full and active a life as possible.

Employment

Unemployment is a problem for many people with epilepsy. A survey in Doncaster in 1996 found that only one-fifth of adults with epilepsy were in employment [43]. There are many possible reasons for this. Sometimes it is because poor seizure control makes some work impractical, e.g. for reasons of safety. At times, it can be the result of an individual's lack of motivation or poor educational or skills attainment. And, of course, failure to find employment may be due to a lack of understanding or even prejudice in a potential employer.

It is important to be positive; up to 70–80% of newly diagnosed cases can expect control by medication. If an individual's seizures are controlled or predictable, most careers should be open, subject to ability and qualifications.

Although most careers should be possible, some are barred, and guidance about prospects of employment for children and young people with epilepsy is needed early. This helps to keep goals for future employment realistic, and reduces the risk of disappointment later. People with epilepsy cannot, for example, become airline pilots, join the Royal Navy or Fire Service or emigrate to certain countries, e.g. Australia. Epilepsy is not necessarily a bar to nursing; each authority sets its own standards. The police will not recruit those with current seizures, and those with a past history are dealt with on an individual basis. Teachers in state schools who develop epilepsy may be barred from teaching physical education, craft, science and home economics. Applicants to teaching must be free of seizures for 2 years. Restrictions exist for any employment involving driving (see page 116). If career advice is needed while the young person with epilepsy is still at college, the local careers advisory service should be contacted. If they are unable to help, the local Training and Enterprise Council might.

Encouragement and advice are needed for those seeking employment. The Disablement Employment Adviser may be able to provide employment advice and help with employment and training courses, and can be contacted through local job centres. Leaflets produced by the epilepsy associations provide good advice about choosing suitable work and clear guidance about how to go about it. Being honest about having epilepsy is stressed as the best route in the long run. A letter from a GP can be very helpful in saying how frequent attacks are, how they affect the individual, and what effect they may have on ability to work. Some employers argue that their insurance would not cover an accident at work. In fact, provided a job has been chosen carefully with full consideration, employers can be reassured that they are covered by normal liability insurance.

For those developing epilepsy while in work, telling an employer may be difficult and there may be an understandable temptation to conceal the fact, but honesty is best. How the information is conveyed is important, and information both about epilepsy in general (obtained from one of the epilepsy association), and specific information about how the individual is affected, may be helpful.

If there are difficulties with employers, and personal negotiation appears to be failing, help may be sought from a trade union, an epilepsy association or local Disablement Employment Adviser. If it comes to the worst, the Disability Discrimination Act may help. The terms of the Disability Discrimination Act (DDA) mean that employers must make reasonable adjustment to the work of people with disabilities or medical conditions where necessary. People with epilepsy are covered by this Act. The DDA also covers recruitment issues. Contact one of the epilepsy associations for further details.

Education

Most children with epilepsy are able to go to a normal school and will rarely have problems with seizures in school time. A minority of children will have difficult epilepsy, often associated with other neurological problems such as learning disability, and will require special residential schooling (see Appendix 1, 'Sources of Help and Advice'). In between are a small group who will be able to attend a normal school with some help. Where a child appears to have special educational needs which a school has difficulty in meeting, the local education authority has to make a Statutory Assessment, and then draw up a Statement of Special Educational Needs. This describes all the child's needs and special help required. Help can often then be provided in the child's ordinary school.

Children are sometimes kept off school after a seizure, because parents fear another seizure happening at school. Some types of absence seizure go unnoticed at school. A combination of seizures, sedation through medication and missing school can cause a child to fall behind educationally. The child may feel under pressure to catch up, resulting in further seizures. Teachers as well as parents should be educated in the problems of children with epilepsy, and teachers made aware of the subtle nature of absence seizures. Children with epilepsy may still have undue restrictions placed on them in sporting and other activities. Parents should be urged to discuss a child's problems with his or her teachers. A letter from the GP explaining the nature of a child's epilepsy, any particular needs and what the child should be able to do can often work wonders.

Where Epilepsy Liaison Sisters are available, they can visit schools on behalf of individual pupils, sort out misunderstandings and provide short talks and videos for teaching staff and pupils.

Driving

To have a single seizure or to develop epilepsy can be devastating for an adult who relies upon being allowed to drive. To be prevented from driving is disappointing for teenagers eagerly approaching the age of 17 years. Coping with modern life without the motor car is too much for many, and not surprisingly some with uncontrolled epilepsy continue to drive and undoubtedly many accidents ensue.

Legislation attempts to balance the risks of a person with epilepsy driving against the psychological and social disadvantages to that person if prevented from doing so. The Driving and Vehicle Licensing Agency (DVLA) has a medical department to consider applications for licences, and also has a medical advisory panel which reviews individual cases (Fig. 8.2). The GP may be asked for medical details but is spared involvement in decisions.

It is important that doctors dealing with patients with epilepsy are fully aware of the driving regulations. Drivers or potential licence applicants who develop epilepsy must be told that, by law, they are prohibited from driving. Anyone experiencing a seizure or developing epilepsy should be told that the law requires that he or she inform the DVLA promptly. It must

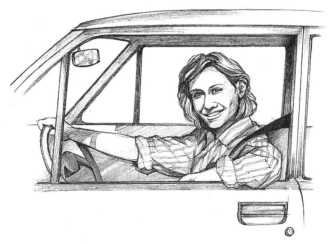

Fig. 8.2 Epilepsy and driving.

be pointed out that it is the personal responsibility of the individual to do this and not the doctor's. Since continuing to drive will be illegal, this may invalidate insurance cover. It is advisable to keep a written record of the information given. **If efforts to persuade a patient to inform the DVLA and surrender a licence fail, a doctor may have to consider disclosure.**

The current driving regulations (revised August 1994)

Group 1 licences (for motor cars and motorcycles). The general intention is to grant ordinary driving licences to those with epilepsy who have been free from any seizures for a whole year, with or without treatment, or have only had attacks during sleep over 3 years. A licence may be granted if the following conditions are satisfied:

1 He or she shall have been completely free from any epileptic attack for a period of 1 year; or

2 In the case of an applicant who has epileptic attack(s) only while asleep, shall have demonstrated a sleep-only pattern for 3 years or more, without attacks while awake;

3 The driving of a vehicle is not likely to be a danger to the public.

Condition (3) may be relevant where other features, such as drug effects, or associated neurological or neuropsychiatric conditions, may affect the ability to drive safely.

Group 2 licences (for large goods vehicles and passenger-carrying vehicles over 3.5 tonnes, and eight seats or more, for hire or reward). An applicant for a licence shall satisfy the following conditions:

1 No epileptic attacks have occurred in the previous 10 years and the sufferer has taken no anti-epileptic drug treatment during this period;

2 There is no continuing liability to epileptic seizures.

The purpose of condition (2) is to exclude persons (whether they have ever experienced seizures or not) who have a brain lesion which might lead to epilepsy, or have a continuing liability to seizures.

The regulations apply whatever the type of seizure, not just tonic–clonic seizures, and so include even very minor disturbances such as a simple partial seizure (even an aura), absence attacks or myoclonic jerks.

Other considerations are as follows.

Single seizures. These are not considered as 'epilepsy' unless a continuing liability can be shown. The DVLA driving law would still apply. (The DVLA usually bans driving for 12 months.)

Provoked seizures. In some circumstances seizures may be provoked (acute symptomatic). The DVLA should still be informed, but where the provocation is unlikely to recur, driving may be allowed at an earlier date. Decisions to allow driving where seizures are related to alcohol or drug abuse are made less readily.

Seizures during treatment changes. The GP or specialist should advise that driving should cease for anything up to 6 months after cessation of anti-epileptic drug treatment. Should a seizure occur during this time the epilepsy driving regulations would apply.

Electroencephalograph changes. These are not usually a bar to driving. The exception is that 3 Hz spike–wave discharges of primary generalized epilepsy are regarded as seizures.

Advice to doctors about driving and epilepsy is available from the Driving and Vehicle Licensing Agency, Swansea SA99 1TU, the epilepsy associations and in Taylor, J.F. (ed.) *Medical Aspects of Fitness to Drive*, published by The Medical Commission on Accident Prevention, 35–43 Lincoln's Inn Fields, London WC2A 3PN.

Sport and leisure

Restrictions should be sensible. Cycling is usually permissible, but a helmet should be worn. Swimming is reasonable if someone with life-saving skills is available and informed (Fig. 8.3). Rock climbing is perhaps best avoided, but most sports and games should be allowed and encouraged.

Sexuality

Sexual problems may arise from the epilepsy itself, from the effects of anti-epileptic medication, and psychological factors including depression and anxiety. Poor self-esteem or limited social opportunities can also play a part. The problems can be divided into two main components—desire and arousal.

Both sexual desire and sexual arousal can be affected to some extent in both sexes in epilepsy. The majority of women with epilepsy appear to have normal sex lives, although both desire and arousal may be inhibited. Men appear to have more problems, more so with arousal than desire, which may be due to epilepsy-related changes in hypothalamic endocrine function. Both epilepsy and some anti-epileptic drugs affect hormones such as prolactin, raised levels of which can affect arousal in men. There is no significant evidence that this leads to any impairment of sexual response in women. Diminished libido and arousal may result from anti-epileptic medication, especially barbiturates.

The fear of having a seizure while making love can have an inhibiting effect in both sexes.

Many are helped by the explanation that problems with sexual arousal are not uncommon in epilepsy or that drugs might be to blame—this often leads to tremendous relief that problems are not due to personal inadequacy.

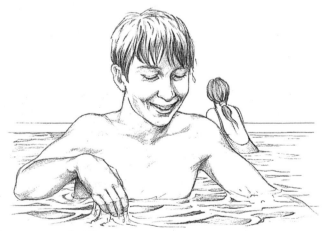

Fig. 8.3 Swimming and epilepsy.

Individual and/or couple psychotherapy can help and may be available through the NHS or Relate.

Contraception

Odd ideas abound, even among doctors and nurses. There is a common misconception that the pill makes epilepsy worse, and another that it interferes with anti-epileptic drugs. Both are mistaken. There is no reason why women with epilepsy taking anti-epileptic medication should not take oral contraceptives. See Chapter 7, pages 95–96, for a full discussion.

Pregnancy and preconceptual counselling

Most women with epilepsy can expect a normal pregnancy, without any increase in seizures, and have a healthy child. However, there is a slightly increased risk of complications and malformations associated with epilepsy itself. See Chapter 7, pages 96–98, for a full discussion.

Inheritance

If the epilepsy is acquired, i.e. the result of injury or infection, the risk of inheriting epilepsy is small, and no different to the rest of the population, that is $1:200$. The risk is greater if there is a strong family history, especially if on both sides. For one parent with idiopathic epilepsy, the risk is approximately $1:30$. The risk of inheritance is greater in some rarer syndromes and in some families, supporting the existence of a genetic tendency in some epilepsies. A specialist opinion may be needed to give an estimate of risk.

Immunization

Past concern has related to the risks of pertussis immunization in three groups of children: those with a close family history of epilepsy, those with a history of febrile convulsions, and those with neonatal brain damage. However, the present view is that children in these categories can be safely immunized against pertussis.

Health and safety in the home

The following advice should be given.

Water is a potential hazard. Patients should never take a bath when alone in the house. When taking a bath, it is advisable to have only a few inches of water in the bath and not to get into the bath with the water still running. Towels may be wrapped around the taps to prevent injury. If seizures are frequent, others in the house should be told that a bath is being taken and the bathroom door should be left unlocked. A shower is a safer alternative. Parents with epilepsy should *never* bath the baby when alone, and it may be best to bath the baby with the bath on the floor rather than on a table.

Patients should be advised to turn pan handles away when cooking, so that pans cannot be knocked over accidentally. A cooker guard improves safety. If attacks are frequent, plates should be taken to the cooker rather than hot pans and dishes to the table. If a microwave is available, it is safer to heat one hot drink, leaving it to cool before taking it out, rather than pouring boiling water into a cup. Irons can be dangerous.

Carrying hot water or hot fat is a common cause of accidents. Those with open fires, gas fires or electric fires with exposed elements should be advised to buy a fireguard that will not readily be knocked over during a seizure.

Glass is dangerous—glass doors and coffee tables should be replaced. Soft pillows should be avoided by those subject to nocturnal seizures (safety pillows are available by mail order). Other hazards include long flexes. Climbing to clean windows, decorating, etc., should be avoided.

Smokers should avoid smoking alone indoors, especially in bed, and should perhaps invest in flame-resistant furnishings and fabrics.

Advice about safety in the home is available from local gas and electricity boards, the Royal Society for the Prevention of Accidents and the epilepsy associations.

About anti-epileptic drugs

Patients, relatives and carers need to have some idea of how drugs work so that they can understand that a regular dose is needed to keep adequate levels in the brain, and recognize and report side-effects.

Taking medication regularly without fail is a difficult discipline. For those with mild epilepsy, forgetting to take a tablet may not matter much, but for those with severe epilepsy it can be very serious. Many patients with poorly controlled epilepsy are, for one reason or another, simply not taking medication regularly and effectively. Epilepsy specialist nurses find that explanation, close support and inventiveness can usually overcome the difficulties, often with dramatic improvement in control.

The simpler the regimen, the better. Most patients can be treated satisfactorily with a twice-daily dosage of the main anti-epileptic drugs, and although many recently diagnosed patients are managed in this way, patients put on medication in the past (or put on medication recently by clinicians living in the past), may be on unnecessarily complicated regimens (see Chapter 5, page 59, for changing and simplifying medication).

Specific points

The following points should be noted.
- Forgetting tablets can swiftly lead to loss of control.
- A plan of action is needed to assist the memory, e.g. simply putting the tablets beside the toothbrush. Patients and relatives should be encouraged to work out a system.
- A pill wallet is useful, or the patient can simply put the day's tablets out and then can see at a glance if a tablet has been forgotten.
- If a dose is forgotten, it should be taken as soon as the mistake is realized, but avoid taking a 'double dose' of carbamazepine.
- If a dose is vomited within a short time, say half an hour, the dose should be repeated when the patient is able to take it.

Living with Epilepsy: 100 Common Questions and Answers 9

When patients with established epilepsy are invited to comment, it is a stark fact that many deny ever having been offered much in the way of information or explanation, or of having felt that they were allowed an opportunity to ask questions. The more determined among them report having had to obtain information for themselves from public libraries or the epilepsy associations.

The following are questions commonly asked by patients, relatives, carers and professionals and have been contributed to by the British Epilepsy Association, the Epilepsy Association of Scotland, Neuroeducation, the University of Birmingham Seizure Clinic and Liaison Service and the Doncaster Epilepsy Specialist Nursing Service.

About epilepsy

1 What is epilepsy and what happens in my brain when a seizure occurs?

In brief, it is useful to use the analogy of electrical activity. Illustrations such as Figs 3.1, 3.2 and 3.4 are useful. See also Chapter 8, page 112.

2 What causes epilepsy? 3 Why did *I* develop seizures?

These questions are closely linked. The reasons behind the question may need exploring. Patients and relatives are mostly concerned with what has caused their own epilepsy. Many assume that epilepsy is a single entity. Some are seeking reassurance that they are not to blame in some way, e.g. inheritance, smoking in pregnancy, agreeing to the immunization of a child against pertussis. For the generally curious, Chapter 2 provides more information about causes. Otherwise see Chapter 8.

4 Can epilepsy be prevented?

Again, the reasons behind the question may require exploration. Everything depends upon what the underlying cause is. Obviously, epilepsy from acquired damage to the brain (e.g. following stroke, intranatal insult or head injury) is potentially preventable.

5 What is my prognosis? 6 Does epilepsy get worse with age? 7 Will my child grow out of epilepsy?

The answers for the individual obviously depend upon the underlying cause. See Chapter 8. Most can be given an encouraging prognosis. For the many patients whose epilepsy will remit, epilepsy can obviously be said to improve with age. Some patients with chronic, resistant epilepsy may deteriorate, but most patients, even those with incomplete control, do not get markedly worse.

8 Can epilepsy be cured?

The only real cure is by surgery for those patients who are suitable, mainly some of those with partial epilepsy arising from a focus which can be safely operated upon. Surgery in epilepsy is covered in Chapter 5.

9 Do seizures cause brain damage?

For most people with epilepsy, there is no evidence that seizures cause permanent brain damage. However, very frequent convulsive seizures can cause damage, especially if prolonged, e.g. status epilepticus. Relatives and carers of patients who have had episode(s) of status epilepticus should be briefed to act quickly to get medical assistance in any future seizures which are prolonged, e.g. beyond 10 minutes. Head injuries associated with seizures can also lead to damage.

10 Is epilepsy life-threatening? Could I die (choke) in a seizure?

The honest answer has to be 'yes' to both questions, but softened by adding 'very rarely'. The overall mortality is two to four times that of the population without epilepsy. The excess mortality is highest among children and young adults. This includes not just accidents associated with seizures but also suicide and sudden unexpected death. The need to take sensible precautions without being overprotected should be stressed.

11 Why aren't my seizures controlled yet?

There may be a variety of reasons. The patient may have severe drug-resistant epilepsy, in which surgery may be a consideration. There may be worsening of an underlying cause. Treatment with anti-epileptic drugs may be inadequate or even inappropriate for the seizure type. (e.g. juvenile myoclonic epilepsy being treated with the wrong anti-epileptic drug; see Case study 2, Chapter 3, page 30). The patient may not be taking his or her medication regularly. The patient may not have epilepsy but some other seizure disorder (see Chapter 4).

12 Could I harm anyone during a seizure?

Part of the mythology to be debunked; most of those asking this question are seeking reassurance. The answer is: 'unusual, and unlikely'. Obviously, a jerking limb might contact a bystander accidentally, and a few patients with complex partial seizures with post-ictal automatism can be confused and aggressive after a seizure.

13 Could I have a seizure making love?

The answer has to be 'of course', but that it would 'not be dangerous'. It is reasonable to say that it is not so very likely, because seizures are less likely when people are active, concentrating and enjoying themselves, which is presumably the case. I suspect that few ask doctors this particular question, possibly because of embarrassment or lack of opportunity. A major concern might be the likely effect on a (patient's) partner who is unaware of what might happen. Certainly, the fear of having a seizure while making love causes anxiety in both men and women with epilepsy and this can affect arousal, in men particularly.

14 Could the symptoms I am experiencing be epileptic in nature?

Some patients do present suspecting that they might have epilepsy. Chapter 4 deals fully with the problems of differential diagnosis. In patients with established epilepsy, it is not uncommon for some to find that they are having more than one seizure manifestation, e.g. a patient with tonic–clonic seizures may begin to recognize simple partial or complex partial attacks, or (if the underlying syndrome is primary generalized epilepsy) absence and myoclonic attacks.

15 I don't have convulsions in a seizure, so is it epilepsy?

It could be. Many seizure types, e.g. absence attacks, simple and complex partial seizures, do not involve convulsive movements. The terms 'fit', 'convulsion' and 'seizure' are all used to describe epileptic attacks. Using the term 'seizure' as a preference avoids confusion.

16 What tests are involved in the diagnosis of epilepsy?
17 Will tests 'prove' whether I have epilepsy or not?

Patients expect tests. Not surprisingly they, like some doctors, expect tests to prove or disprove the diagnosis. Patients should be helped to understand the reasons for the different tests and what to expect. Most patients these days will have an electroencephalogram (EEG), possibly a computed tomography (CT) scan, and an increasing number will have magnetic resonance imaging (MRI), particularly if they have partial seizures. Leaflets are available and usually provide the following information.

EEG test

An EEG records electrical activity in the brain. It helps in the diagnosis, but like other tests does not itself 'prove' epilepsy. The EEG test is painless and is carried out by a technician who will explain what is going to happen. The patient lies down. Up to 20 small pads or electrodes are placed on the head and either stuck down with glue or held in place with a cap. The electrodes are connected by wires to the EEG machine. The patient is asked to keep still, and then asked to do a number of things: open and close the eyes, take deep breaths for a few minutes and look at a flashing light. The whole procedure lasts 30–60 minutes. The main complaint people have is about having to wash the glue out of their hair afterwards. The EEG is reported on later by a specialist, so there may be a delay before the result is known.

An 'ambulatory' EEG may be needed to try to find out what happens electrically during a seizure. The patient is able to walk around, and has a tape recorder strapped to the waist.

CT scan

CT is a special way of X-raying the brain in 'slices', and builds up a picture of the structure of the brain. It may show up an underlying cause of epilepsy. The CT scan is sometimes called a CAT scan, which is an abbreviation for computed axial tomography. The procedure is not painful and involves lying down with the head in an opening. Sometimes an injection is given into an arm vein to improve the contrast.

MRI

MRI is being used more, particularly when surgery is being considered. It provides very detailed images of the brain structure. However, it cannot prove the diagnosis of epilepsy either. It is expensive, not painful, but noisy, and since the patient has to be enclosed it can be frightening for small children, who may require an anaesthetic to keep them still.

18 How often should I see my specialist?

Everyone is different. Usually, this should be agreed with the specialist. Most patients will only continue to see a specialist if seizures and treatment involve problems that the specialist can help with. Most patients are discharged to GP care once control appears satisfactory. Patients and/or parents should be advised to report any worsening in control, changes in seizures, the development of drug side-effects or new symptoms to their GP, so that he or she can decide whether they should return to see a specialist.

19 Why have I developed epilepsy so late in life?

Late-onset epilepsy is almost always 'partial epilepsy' and due to a focal lesion. The most common cause is cerebrovascular, but tumours, which are usually metastatic, are also an important cause. Patients are not always as reassured as we might expect them to be if told that their epilepsy is due to 'hardening of the arteries', because of fears of dementia. Epilepsy in the elderly is covered fully in Chapter 7.

20 My memory is poor. Is this because of my epilepsy or anti-epileptic drugs?

In children, recurrent absence attacks can appear to impair memory, simply because they have missed what has been going on. Frequent severe seizures can lead to loss of memory both around and during the seizures. If the underlying cerebral function is poor or deteriorating this can also affect memory.

Anti-epileptic drugs are the main cause of reduced mental functioning, including memory. These drugs vary in their effects. Polytherapy is particularly prone to cause problems. The newer drugs promise to have fewer side-effects (see Chapters 5 and 6).

21 Can I stop a seizure happening once my aura has begun?

Some people can stave off a seizure by using a variety of methods such as concentrating on something else, by relaxation training, biofeedback and even aromatherapy. Some patients will report having been able to do the opposite, i.e. induce a seizure, even admitting to using this ability to get out of something they did not want to do.

22 What should we do when our child has a tonic–clonic seizure?

See 'First aid and what to do' in Chapter 8, page 112.

23 When should I give my child rectal diazepam?

The source of this question is commonly a parent phoning for advice having been supplied with a prescription, misunderstanding or forgetting the instructions, or worse, not receiving any. This preparation is mainly used for febrile convulsions, but occasionally for children prone to prolonged epileptic seizures. The point of including this question is to emphasize the importance of providing adequate instructions. In this case, the use of the drug should be demonstrated (short of injecting it), perhaps by a nurse. 'When' is best made clear by written instructions, e.g. if an attack is prolonged for more than 5 or 10 minutes.

24 When should I call an ambulance after a seizure has started?

An ambulance or medical help is not usually necessary, unless the seizure is prolonged for more than 10 minutes, or if there are repeated seizures or if an injury has occurred.

25 My child may need rectal diazepam at school—do the teachers have to administer this, as they seem reluctant?

Teachers may not be allowed to give rectal diazepam. Teachers find themselves in a difficult situation: they are concerned about their legal position and there are practical difficulties about how and where to do it. Sometimes the school nurse or matron, if available, will administer the drug. It is necessary in any case that the school has specific instructions for its use. It may be that, if frequent administration is necessary, a mainstream school may not be advisable.

26 Is epilepsy infectious?

Well, we know that it is not infectious. But it is a question that gets asked, and it is not unknown for neighbours to prevent their children playing with a child with epilepsy because they 'know that it is catching'.

Precipitating factors

27 Will different foods or drinks trigger seizures?

Some people are convinced that certain foods trigger seizures, but there is little evidence for this. Some (especially those who suffer migraine) claim that foods which trigger their migraine can also trigger a seizure. Aspartate in fizzy drinks is one of the substances said to trigger seizures, although there is no research to fully support this.

28 Does stress bring on seizures?

Yes, it can, however, stress is part of life and, realistically, it cannot be avoided. Manipulating relatives to avoid stressful situations must be discouraged. Stress management and relaxation therapy can help some patients quite a lot, and may be available locally.

29 Does exercise bring on seizures?

Quite the opposite. Being active both physically and mentally is helpful. Boredom is more likely to lead to seizures, particularly if this involves dozing off in those prone to sleep seizures.

30 Can alcohol trigger seizures?

It is important to remember that alcohol can induce seizures in people who do not have epilepsy, usually a withdrawal seizure after a binge. Large amounts of alcohol can trigger seizures. It is not uncommon for patients to leave off anti-epileptic medication when intending to imbibe, for example at a wedding, because of the usual warning on the label on the prescribed medication 'Not to be taken with alcohol'. It can prove to be a mistake.

Drinking in moderation (taken together with the tablets) seems the best solution for most patients.

Other medical aspects

31 Can I pass my epilepsy on to my children?

Briefly, there is only a very slightly increased risk in most cases. Genetic counselling may be indicated when there is a strong family history. See Chapter 8, page 120.

32 I have epilepsy. Can I have children, i.e. conceive?

Epilepsy can have an effect on fertility and so can the drugs, however, this is rarely a problem for most women with epilepsy. There is a high incidence of menstrual irregularity in women with partial seizures of temporal lobe origin. There is also a higher incidence of polycystic ovary syndrome, possibly even greater in women on sodium valproate. Perhaps the questioner may be wondering whether she should have children, as in Question 31.

33 Will epilepsy affect my physical or emotional development?

There in no reason why having epilepsy should affect physical development in someone who has no physical disability to start with. That is, apart from injuries associated with seizures. Treatment with phenytoin can have cosmetic side-effects such as coarsening of the skin and hirsutism, and some other anti-epileptic drugs cause weight gain. There is no doubt that many individuals do suffer psychological and emotional problems, but this is felt to be a consequence of having epilepsy, not something that is a component of epilepsy. The answer is, 'It can, but it doesn't have to'.

34 Will epilepsy affect my sex life?

It shouldn't necessarily, however, both sexual desire and sexual arousal can be affected to some extent in both sexes in epilepsy, but most women have normal sex lives. Men have more of a problem with arousal than desire, which may be due to epilepsy-related changes in hypothalamic endocrine function. Some anti-epileptic drugs affect hormones, which can affect arousal in men, but there is no significant evidence that this leads to any impairment of sexual response in women. Both epilepsy and its treatment can alter the menstrual cycle and affect fertility (see Chapter 7, page 95).

Many are helped by the explanation that problems with sexual arousal are not uncommon in epilepsy—this often leads to tremendous relief that it is not due to personal inadequacy. Individual and/or couple psychotherapy can help.

35 Should my child have pertussis and/or measles/mumps/rubella (MMR) vaccines as I have a history of epilepsy?

For a time, there was uncertainty about the risks of pertussis immunization causing epilepsy in these and other circumstances, but now it is considered safe. The advice should be that irrespective of a personal or close family history the vaccine should be given.

36 Do I need to take my medication while pregnant?
37 Will the anti-epileptic medication affect the foetus?

The decision whether or not to continue treatment has to be based upon the risks of recurrent seizures if the patient has control, or of the seizures worsening. These issues need to be considered well before pregnancy is decided upon. Most of the main anti-epileptic drugs may have effects on the foetus, but usually by the time pregnancy is reported these will have occurred, and it will probably be best to continue with treatment. See Chapter 7 on preconceptual counselling and epilepsy in pregnancy.

38 Can I breast-feed my baby while taking medication?

Yes. The baby will receive less anti-epileptic drug in breast milk than when in the womb. It is advisable to take safety measures when feeding like sitting on the floor, particularly if not seizure-free (Fig. 9.1).

39 Is epilepsy affected by hormonal changes?
40 My seizures are period-related. Will they stop when I go through the menopause?

Yes, epilepsy can be affected by hormonal changes. Some women who already have epilepsy, particularly if seizures are related to the menstrual cycle, *may* find that their epilepsy stops after the menopause. Hormone replacement therapy at the menopause is quite a good idea for women on anti-epileptic drugs, which cause calcium deficiency, but may sometimes lead to an increase in seizure frequency.

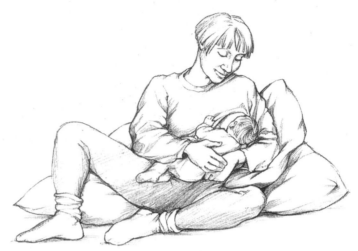

Fig. 9.1 Breast-feeding and epilepsy.

Medication and other treatment

41 Do I have to take anti-epileptic medication all my life?

It is not possible to predict accurately who is likely to be able to stop treatment without the risk of seizures recurring. Most people starting with epilepsy can be told that if they gain control with anti-epileptic drugs, they may stand a good chance of coming off treatment in a few years, but that it should not be considered for at least 2 or 3 years. The following factors make the likelihood of seizures recurring more likely: age over 16 years, taking more than one anti-epileptic drug, experiencing seizures after starting anti-epileptic drugs, a history of tonic–clonic seizures (both primary and secondarily generalized), myoclonic seizures and an abnormal EEG.

42 Am I taking the right dosage of medication?

Table 5.2 (page 54) gives the dosage ranges for adults and Table 7.2 (page 90) the ranges for children. The 'right dose' will vary and should be that which is sufficient to control seizures and not that which produces so-called satisfactory serum levels. Provided the patient is taking the tablets, the best measurement is how the patient is.

43 Do I have to pay for my prescriptions?

No, not in the UK, but you must get the appropriate form filled in and sent to the local Health Authority, or in Scotland the Health Board, in order to get exemption. The form is available from the GP, pharmacies or a local hospital.

44 What should I do if I forget to take my anti-epileptic medication?

Ideally seek medical advice, but if this is not possible, the short answer is to take the dose as soon as the error is realized, but avoid taking a double dose in the case of carbamazepine because of side-effects, e.g. delay the next dose slightly.

45 I am very forgetful about taking my tablets three times a day. I tend to forget the afternoon dose. What can I do about this?

A doctor must first consider whether it is necessary for the treatment to be taken three times a day. Most standard preparations can be effective in twice-daily dosage and slow-release preparations may be tried (see Chapters 5 and 6). To prompt memory, consider something like a pill wallet or watch alarm. See also Chapter 8.

46 Can I get used to a drug so that it no longer has any effect?

This is not likely, although some individuals develop tolerance to some drugs. The levels of active drug can vary in an individual in some circumstances such as pregnancy and after marked changes in weight. If seizures become more frequent without any change in the dose or administration of medication, the patient should be reviewed.

47 What are the side-effects of my medication?
48 What are the long-term effects of anti-epileptic drugs?
49 I have put on a lot of weight. Is this due to my medication?

For full answers to these three questions, consult the section on individual anti-epileptic drugs in Chapter 6, individual drug data sheets or the *British National Formulary*. Many patients are supplied with this and other information with their prescriptions.

In brief, more common side-effects are as follows. Most first- and second-line anti-epileptic drugs will cause some sedation and can cause giddiness. Phenytoin is renowned for its cosmetic effects and gingival hypertrophy. Sodium valproate, and to a lesser extent carbamazepine and oxcarbazepine, can cause weight gain. Sodium valproate can cause hair thinning, which is reversible.

If side-effects are being discussed, it is probably prudent to record that the information has been given, particularly to record any advice to consult for preconceptual counselling.

50 Are my drugs addictive?

There is no evidence that anti-epileptic drugs are addictive, although dependency on benzodiazepines such as clobazam might theoretically be possible.

51 I always feel tired and sleepy—is this normal?

Epilepsy does not cause sleepiness except sometimes immediately after a seizure. Anti-epileptic drug medication certainly can, and may be a reason for changing to another drug or a change of formulation of a current drug, e.g. to a sustained-release preparation.

52 Do the drugs lower my sexual drive?

Very occasionally they may, but it is difficult to be certain because sexual problems are common in people in general. Some anti-epileptic drugs affect hormones which can affect arousal in men, but there is no significant evidence that this leads to any impairment of sexual response in women. In men, diminished libido and arousal may result from anti-epileptic medication, especially barbiturates. The explanation that drugs might be to blame will often bring relief that the problem is not due to personal inadequacy. Individual and/or couple psychotherapy can help.

53 My doctor prescribed Epilim, but the chemist gave me sodium valproate—is this OK?

Technically speaking, they are the same drug, but sodium valproate is supplied in its 'generic' form by several manufacturers. As a consequence, there may be some variation in how it is absorbed by the body. It might not make any difference, but all epilepsy experts consider that it is safer for an individual to continue on the same preparation of any anti-epileptic drug. This can only be ensured by prescribing by brand. The advice would be to ask the prescriber to ensure that this continued to happen.

54 What is monotherapy?

Monotherapy is of course treatment with one drug only, but the questioner may think it is a new treatment.

55 How often should I have blood tests?

No wonder patients get confused. Some epileptologists do anti-epileptic drug serum levels all the time, particularly if they come from a pharmacological background. Other epileptologists, usually neurologists, will say through gritted teeth that they are rarely needed. Obstetricians feel that they have to do them. GPs have come to believe that their audit results are poor if they are shown not to have done them. Patients expect them. The fashionable answer is 'hardly ever'. Serum levels are useful to check on compliance, useful if drug toxicity is suspected and useful to help adjust the dose of phenytoin specifically.

56 Will the anti-epileptic medication be all right together with other treatment which my doctor gives me?

The more common interactions are outlined in Chapter 6, and more extensive information is provided in the *British National Formulary*. It in doubt, the information pharmacist in the local hospital may be able to help answer specific queries.

57 Can I take 'over-the-counter' medicines as well as my anti-epileptic medication?

Few 'over-the-counter' remedies are likely to conflict with anti-epileptic drugs, but patients should be advised to tell the community pharmacist about the drugs they are taking when they are considering purchasing 'over-the-counter' medicines.

58 Now that I am on anti-epilepsy drugs, can I still drink alcohol?

See Question 30 on epilepsy and alcohol. In brief, yes, in moderation, and do not leave off your tablets when you intend to drink.

59 Can I take the contraceptive pill or have the three-monthly injection with my anti-epileptic drugs?

Briefly, yes, but you may need a higher dose of the pill with some enzyme-inducing anti-epileptic drugs, and the three-monthly injection may need to be given more frequently. See a full discussion in 'Epilepsy in women', Chapter 7, pages 95–96.

60 Will I be able to have hormone replacement therapy if I am on medication for my epilepsy?

Yes, it might even protect against the tendency of some anti-epileptic drugs to cause calcium loss. However, sometimes hormone replacement therapy can lead to an increase in seizures, quite unrelated to the anti-epileptic drugs.

61 Is there a special diet which could help my epilepsy?

Special diet has little to offer most patients with epilepsy. Ketogenic diets are the only dietary measures with any success in epilepsy. They are only used in a few special centres, mainly for children with some forms of epilepsy, and have no application for most people with epilepsy. They have a high fat content and are very unpalatable.

62 Could I have surgery for epilepsy?

Surgery to cure or improve control is used increasingly year by year. It is only used in people in whom drugs have proved unsuccessful. It is mainly used for removing parts of the brain responsible for the onset of seizures, and to a lesser extent for dividing nerve connections. Facilities do not yet exist to offer investigations and operations for all those who might benefit. The investigations are themselves very rigorous. For further details see Chapter 5.

63 I have tried all of the different drugs, and now I've been told that I do not have a 'focus', and so cannot have surgery. What next?

Inevitably, not everyone is suitable for surgery, nor capable of being controlled by drugs. There may be nothing else to offer, and it may be unkind to offer alternatives which are unlikely to help. Alternatives are raised in some of the following questions.

64 Could I have the new vagal implant?

A vagal implant is an interesting new treatment consisting of a device implanted to stimulate the vagal nerve. It is said to have a success rate equivalent to new drugs. The procedure is simple and safe, and now available on the NHS. See also Chapter 5.

65 Are there any alternative/complementary treatments that are successful in controlling or curing epilepsy? 66 Does hypnotherapy/aromatherapy, etc. help? 67 What is biofeedback?

A number of alternative treatments are used with varying success, but are not widely available and are not generally a substitute for anti-epileptic drugs, but they may help. Any therapy, such as relaxation therapy or stress management, which can promote relaxation is likely to help. Work at the Birmingham Seizure Clinic suggests that aromatherapy can help to control seizures in some patients. Behavioural therapy can be used to avoid seizure-provoking situations, e.g. photic stimulation, distracting activity during an aura. Biofeedback is a technique which involves the individual learning to control their own EEG activity. In this country, work on biofeedback has been mainly carried out by Professor P. Fenwick at the Maudsley Hospital, London.

For more detail on alternative treatments, see Chapter 5.

Lifestyle implications

68 What are the driving regulations for epilepsy and ordinary licences? 69 What are the driving regulations for epilepsy and LGV/PCV licences?

The current driving regulations are covered extensively in Chapter 8, page 116.

Briefly, the intention is to allow ordinary licences to those with epilepsy who have been free from attacks for 1 year, with or without treatment, or who have had at least 3 years with attacks only occurring during sleep. Vocational licences can be granted once there is 'no continued liability to seizures', *and* there have been no attacks for 10 years during which time the individual has been off anti-epileptic drugs.

All licence-holders are required to inform the DVLA if they have any disability (mental or physical) that is likely to affect their fitness as a driver that is expected to last more than 3 months.

70 What should I do about driving if my anti-epileptic medication is withdrawn?

The DVLA recommends that driving be suspended from the start of drug reduction and for 6 months after withdrawal (this is advisory and not a regulation).

71 Is there a motor insurance company who are sympathetic to people with epilepsy?

Yes, there is. Contact one of the epilepsy associations for advice (see 'Sources of Help and Advice', Appendix 1).

72 What jobs can I do with a history of epilepsy?
73 Can I continue with my work after being diagnosed as having epilepsy?
74 Should I tell my (prospective) employer that I have epilepsy?

Employment issues including the very few jobs barred to those with a history of epilepsy are covered in some detail in Chapter 8, page 114. The epilepsy associations provide leaflets and telephone helplines for specific problems. For practical information and tactics for dealing with problems including employment, Chappell, B. and Crawford, P. *Epilepsy at your fingertips.* London: Class Publishing, 1999 is great.

It should be possible to continue in most jobs, and most careers should be possible if an individual's seizures are controlled or predictable. Obviously, jobs involving driving or dangerous situations are likely to be out of the question until it can be shown that the epilepsy is controlled. Some employers will offer alternative employment, and a letter from a doctor or nurse setting out the position can help. Honesty is to be recommended, although it is understandable that some prefer not to disclose that they have epilepsy for fear of discrimination. Most application forms require this information, and direct questions are best answered honestly. Employers need to know under the Health and Safety at Work Act. The best time to raise the issue of epilepsy is towards the end of an interview, by which time the candidate will have done his or her best to sell him or herself. In difficult cases, negotiation is the best way, but if all else fails people with epilepsy are covered by the Disability Discrimination Act (DDA).

75 Will epilepsy affect school work?

It can, but it should not for most children with epilepsy. Frequent seizures of any sort can be disruptive and cause work to be missed. It is important to discuss how to deal with a child's problems with teachers. Keeping a child off school, sending the child home or taking him or her out of class for the rest of the day should be avoided if at all possible. Helpful teachers will attempt to make up for what is missed, whether from tonic–clonic seizures or barely observable absence attacks.

Some school lessons might pose dangers. Practical science lessons involving bunsen burners and chemicals, and domestic science, are obvious examples.

Medication can also affect concentration and may need to be reviewed if there is a problem.

See also Chapter 8, pages 115–116.

76 I think my child may have special educational needs. Where should I go for help?

If the child is under school age, the local education authority (LEA) will help. If the child is over 2 years, the LEA can be asked to make a Statutory Assessment of his or her special educational needs. Even if a child is under 2 years, the LEA may be able to help.

If the child is already in school, the child's teacher or the head teacher should be approached. There will be a teacher in the school with special responsibility for children with special educational needs.

See also Chapter 8, page 116.

77 Can I use a computer, play video games or go to discos?

For individuals who do not have photosensitive epilepsy, the answer is certainly 'yes'. For patients with photosensitive epilepsy, the answer is usually also 'yes', but certain sensible precautions are advisable. See Chapter 8, page 114.

78 How can I help to prevent accidents at home?

It is mainly common sense. See Chapter 8, page 121, for further information.

Sometimes safety can be expensive, for example, replacing an open fire or making other changes. Help may be available from Social Services.

79 Can I smoke?

Smoking has no effect on epilepsy, but if the individual must smoke then thought needs to be given to safety, for example, not smoking indoors alone or in bed ever.

80 Will street drugs affect my epilepsy?

Yes, they may. Some street drugs can cause seizures, as alcohol can. The activities that accompany taking them, such as late nights and lack of sleep, can also make seizures more likely.

81 Can I go swimming/ride a bike/rock climbing/boxing/scuba diving, etc.?

Usually 'yes' to swimming and cycling. It is advisable to inform the pool attendant, and it is a good idea to go swimming with a friend who will watch out for you (the American 'buddy' system). It is best to wear a helmet when cycling. Boxing and contact sports are advised against by most epileptologists. Scuba diving sounds pretty problematical, and the Scuba Diving Association are opposed on the supposed grounds that the depth of water affects anti-epileptic drugs, which sounds odd. Rock climbing is inadvisable.

82 Can a child with epilepsy climb school gym apparatus?

Teachers often ask this. The advice has to be 'no', unless the epilepsy is well controlled, otherwise children should be allowed to use low apparatus and take part in activities which do not involve climbing. As far as outdoor school sports are concerned, throwing the javelin or other objects would be unwise. Advice has to be tailored to the individual child.

83 Can I travel abroad? 84 Can I get my medication abroad?

There is no reason why people with epilepsy should not travel abroad. Medication can be obtained abroad, but it will usually be necessary to see a local doctor. Preparations will usually have different names and may not be absorbed exactly the same. It is best to travel with more medication than is required and to divide it up and keep some separately (in case luggage is lost or stolen). For some countries outside Europe, it may be wise to carry a letter from a doctor specifying the nature and need for medication.

Timing doses may be a problem, and keeping a watch to UK time may be helpful.

85 Can I travel by air?

Yes, but inform the airline when checking in.

86 Do I need extra health insurance while on holiday?

It is advisable. The British Epilepsy Association and other epilepsy associations can provide information about this.

87 Can I use a sun bed?

Yes.

Sources of help or information

88 Which welfare benefits am I entitled to claim because I have epilepsy?

There are a range of benefits available, depending upon the degree of disability and other circumstances. Some of the application forms are formidable, and in order to get across the amount of incapacity or disability caused by an individual's epilepsy, it is advisable to seek assistance in completing them. A Welfare Rights Officer from the Citizen's Advice Bureau or Social Services would be best. There is also a Benefit Enquiry Line (BEL) which specializes in benefits for people with disabilities, call 0800 882200, and a Form Completion Service for ICA, SDA, DWA, DLA and AA, call 0800 441144.

Doctors, nurses and other professionals may be asked for information by the Benefits Agency or by representatives on behalf of an applicant. To help, there are suggestions included in the following outlines about how this might be done.

Free prescriptions

The appropriate form can be obtained from the GP, pharmacist, hospital, Health Authority or Health Board.

Incapacity Benefit

Incapacity Benefit replaced Sickness Benefit and Invalidity Benefit after 13 April 1995. Anyone already on the former benefits was transferred automatically to the new benefit.

Incapacity benefit is not means tested, but is taxable after 28 weeks. There are additional allowances for dependants.

The decision regarding incapacity to work is taken by a 'decision maker' (previously known as an Adjudication Officer) from the Benefits Agency, based upon information provided by the patient on a questionnaire, by the patient's GP, and a medical examination if necessary.

In the first 28 weeks of incapacity, most individuals will be assessed on their ability to do their own job. After that, they will have to undergo a 'personal capability assessment' (previously known as the 'all work' test), unless they have severe mental illness. At 29 weeks, most claimants will be sent a self-assessment questionnaire as a basis for the assessment, and a medical examination may be necessary.

To satisfy the 'personal capability assessment' 15 or more 'points' are required from either physical or mental 'descriptors', or a combination of both. The questionnaire asks about the frequency of 'fits or something like this' but the decision is based, more precisely, upon having 'an involuntary episode of lost or altered consciousness' sufficiently frequently. To get the necessary 15 points on epilepsy alone, the episodes must occur 'at least once a month' (or more frequently). Applicants often report only convulsive seizures and fail to include absence attacks or complex partial seizures, but these count too. If a doctor, nurse or other carer is asked to supply evidence **it is important to include the frequency of all seizure types experienced**.

Job Seekers Allowance

Payable for up to 182 days if actively seeking work and having enough Class 1 National Insurance contributions for the 2 tax years before the current benefit year.

Income Support

This is available if savings are less than £8000, and the applicant is aged 18 years or older, not working 16 hours a week or more and not in full-time non-advanced education. If the patient has a partner, he or she must not be working 24 hours or more a week and must be seeking employment. Savings between £3000 and £8000 are assumed to produce an income. Each block of £250 causes a deduction of £1 off the weekly Income Support.

Disability Living Allowance

This is an allowance for people under 65, who are so disabled that they have needs to do with personal care and/or mobility. This is an important benefit for some with severe epilepsy, and securing it may depend upon the quality of information provided by doctors and others. **Crucial information includes: the types of seizure, severity, frequency, presence of and adequacy of any warning, and post-ictal state**.

Care component. This is available if help is needed with bodily functions or supervision is required to prevent danger to self or others during the day or night. There are three rates, depending on the frequency and length of attention, and amount of supervision. As far as epilepsy is concerned, those with frequent seizures during the day and requiring supervision are likely to qualify for the middle rate. It is likely that a claimant with epilepsy who qualifies for this on the grounds of 'need for supervision' will also qualify for the lower rate mobility component.

Mobility component. This is available for people aged 5 or over. There are two rates. The higher rate is for people virtually unable to walk and this rarely applies to epilepsy. The lower rate, however, is for those able to walk, but who require guidance or supervision 'to avoid substantial danger' when outdoors, and this often applies to those with frequent seizures.

Disability Living Allowance is also available to parents with epilepsy caring for an infant or young child if, in the event of an attack occurring without warning, the parent may drop or fall on the child. In this case, the parent may need supervision during the day, or while walking outdoors. A documented episode of 'spontaneous status epilepticus' may also attract this benefit until the risk of recurrence declines—usually 3 years.

Attendance Allowance

For people over 65 years who require help with bodily functions or supervision to prevent danger to self or others.

Therapeutic earnings

If in receipt of Incapacity Benefit and the GP considers—and Social Security agrees—that some paid work would be therapeutically beneficial.

Severe Disablement Allowance

A weekly cash, tax free benefit paid to people who cannot work because of severe illness or disability and do not have sufficient NI contributions to qualify for Incapacity Benefit. The patient must be aged 16 years or over, and under 65 years, and:
• must have been incapable of working for a continuous period of 28 consecutive weeks because of illness or disability (a medical certificate is required);
• must be resident in the UK;
• if 16, 17 or 18, must not be in full-time education;
• must be assessed as at least 75–80% disabled, or become incapable of work on or before his or her 20th birthday, or passported to the test of 80% disablement.

Council Tax Benefit

The applicant must be 18 years or over and on a low income. People getting Income Support or Income-based Jobseekers Allowance may get all their council tax liability paid. It is reduced by 25% if living alone. The applicant's capital must be no more than £16 000.

Industrial Injuries Disablement Benefit

Disabling epilepsy resulting from an accident at work may attract this benefit.

Disability Working Allowance

A tax-free allowance is paid on top of low wages or self-employed earnings for people whose disabilities put them at a disadvantage in getting a job. To qualify, the applicant must be 16 years or older, live in the UK, normally work 16 hours or more a week and have a physical or mental disability which puts the applicant at a disadvantage. The patient must have been getting one of a range of qualifying benefits in the 8 weeks prior to the claim for this allowance, and the applicant or his/her partner must not have savings or capital of over £16 000.

89 Can I get any help from Social Services?

Provision by Social Service Departments varies, but may include the following:
• warden control and call alarm systems (possible charge);
• home carer, to supervise work or housework, do shopping, ironing or help with washing and dressing;
• meals on wheels;
• Occupational Therapy Assessment for showers, ramps, handrails. (Housing departments carry out alterations such as rehanging doors in bathrooms and toilets.)

90 Can I have an Orange Badge (for parking)?

Yes, if you are receiving the full mobility allowance of the Disability Living Allowance. This also entitles the holder to Vehicle Exemption Duty (VED). The Orange Badge scheme is expected to be replaced by a new Blue Badge, which will be phased in throughout the European Community from April 2000.

91 Can I get reduced rates on public transport?

Epilepsy sufferers are eligible for a Disabled Person's Railcard if 'disabled by recurrent attacks in spite of drug treatment'. The application, on a form supplied by the Association of Train Operating Companies, must be certified by the patient's registered medical practitioner.

A few local authorities subsidize transport for patients with epilepsy, but this is not widespread. Local enquiries are advised.

92 Where can I obtain protective headgear?

This should be available on specialist advice through the local district hospital.

93 Is there an alarm system I can have which will alert my family that a seizure has started?

Some Social Service Departments have local arrangements. Commercial systems are available. Further details are available from the epilepsy associations.

94 Is there a counselling service available for me?
95 Where is the nearest support group for my area?
96 Where is the nearest epilepsy clinic to my home?
97 Where are the nearest assessment centres to my home?
98 We are elderly, our son/daughter has severe epilepsy—where can we get long-term accommodation for him or her?
99 Where can I get identification cards/jewellery?
100 Where can I learn more about epilepsy?

In the absence of local services or advice, information on these questions is best sought through one of the epilepsy associations. See Appendix 1, 'Sources of Help and Advice'.

Improving Services: a Structure for Care 10

In Chapter 1, the history of epilepsy and the development of epilepsy services were traced against a background of social prejudices and difficulties facing those with epilepsy. Also considered were the difficulties which GPs perceive in managing epilepsy, the deficiencies and unmet needs for services and information revealed by audits and surveys, and the potential contribution of general practice.

This chapter develops the theme, suggesting how general practice might set about improving practice-based care, and also influence service development through the commissioning and purchasing process.

Although GPs and primary care teams can do a great deal to provide and improve their own services for patients with epilepsy, there are limits. General practice can only provide satisfactory care within a structure that includes adequate specialist services. Most parts of the UK do not have any form of specialist epilepsy service. What can be done, if you do not have such a service?

Documents such as the 'Epilepsy Needs Document' [7], 'Purchasing and Providing Epilepsy Outpatient Services: A Guide to Good Practice' (Appendix 3), 'Epilepsy Needs Revisited' [8] and more recently a major report by the Clinical Standards Advisory Group (CSAG) *Services for Patients with Epilepsy* [11] are useful and important resources in outlining patient needs and specifying service requirements. They do not, however, provide an immediate picture of what the burden of epilepsy might be for a community, nor indicate what the potential for health gain might be for a particular district or for a general practice. Quite rightly, they advocate what is ideal, but at first sight look to have very expensive implications, particularly for a health authority starting apparently from scratch. Two publications described as tool kits appeared in 1999. One, the *Epilepsy Task Force Service Development Kit* [9], included earlier publications plus useful examples of good practice. The other, from the Epilepsy Advisory Board, *Epilepsy Care—Making it Happen* [10], is very comprehensive and includes a 'tool kit' to plan service development.

Most of the few existing epilepsy services have grown from small beginnings. Below is a description of how one such service was developed in Doncaster.

Case study: the Doncaster Epilepsy Service

In 1987, Doncaster (population 290 000) was calculated to have about 1700 patients with epilepsy; there were about 150 or more new cases each year and 300 or more would be referred with possible epilepsy. A visiting neurologist conducting one general neurology clinic each week saw most adult epilepsy. Children with epilepsy were seen by paediatricians and most chronic epilepsy was in the care of GPs.

Numerous surveys and audits had highlighted inadequacies in care for patients with epilepsy, as well as unmet needs for counselling and information [16–20]. Audits as part of a programme to improve epilepsy care in the author's Doncaster practice [12,13] had confirmed the extent of local need and also shown that considerable improvement could be achieved. Approximately one-quarter of patients with chronic epilepsy had improved seizure control and one-quarter reduced drug side-effects. A tendency to misdiagnose epilepsy was observed in hospital doctors who were not experts in epilepsy. It was argued that there was a need for a local specialist epilepsy service based on an epilepsy clinic.

At a meeting between GPs, the neurologist, general physicians, paediatricians and a British Epilepsy Association representative, it was agreed that a case should be made for a collaborative approach to epilepsy care with an epilepsy clinic and protocols for shared care. The neurologist offered to make over one clinic each month as an epilepsy clinic on the grounds that epilepsy was the most common chronic neurological condition, accounted for about 40% of his outpatient workload and epilepsy clinics had been shown to be more effective [66].

An application to the health authority to fund a clinical assistant to work in the clinic was not immediately successful, but an application to the Primary Care Development Fund for 'start-up funds' was. This provided funds for a clinical assistant/facilitator, guideline development and, most importantly as it subsequently turned out, allowed the creation of the first ever post of community-based specialist Epilepsy Liaison Nurse.

The service, set up in 1988, has proved to be popular and effective [24]. As the service developed, joint funding was provided by the

Family Practitioner Committee and the Health Authority, and later a second full-time specialist nurse was added in 1992.

The service has proved effective in a number of ways. From the outset, previously unrecognized problems of clinical management (compliance, unreported seizures, misunderstanding of treatment) and of coping (at home, school, work) were identified and in many cases resolved. Once clinical management could be supervised and supported in the community, fewer clinic attendances were necessary and safer earlier discharge from the clinic became possible. Establishing liaison with schools, employers and care workers in residential homes for learning disability, and supplying information and support, has provided help for many who could never have benefited from a solely hospital-based service.

Comment

A number of important factors underpinned the success in establishing the epilepsy service in Doncaster. In particular: evidence of local need and potential for health gain; evidence from elsewhere that a special epilepsy clinic was a more effective way of providing care; local support by clinicians who were likely to be affected; the prior existence of some sort of neurology service upon which to build; the presence of individuals willing to take a lead; and finally, perseverance and luck.

Influencing service change through purchasing

The National Health Service (NHS) has changed since the Doncaster service was set up. The power of general practice to influence service provision exercised first through fundholding and through membership of commissioning forums is now likely to be greater through Primary Care Groups (PCGs). PCGs will be able to specify epilepsy services in their contracts and include a requirement for information and counselling. In the new climate of a 'primary care-led NHS', projects which favour a shift of resources from secondary care to primary care can be the flavour of the month, and it should not be overlooked that a community-based specialist epilepsy nurse represents an effective shift in that direction.

In making a case for a new service specifically for epilepsy, purchasers will need to be persuaded of the following:
- that epilepsy is an important common problem;
- that there are many inadequately met health needs to do with epilepsy locally;

- that there is a potential for significant and important health gain;
- that the proposal has been shown to have worked elsewhere;
- that it is not going to cost too much. It should preferably be largely possible from within existing resources, e.g. by re-allocation or reorganization;
- that it will make more effective and efficient use of resources already being spent on epilepsy (electroencephalograms (EEGs), computed tomography (CT) scans and other tests);
- that part of the proposed service (the community-based specialist nurse) involves a significant shift from secondary to primary care.

Progress on these points may persuade an authority to consider additional modest support from 'development monies', and later development will depend upon evidence of effectiveness.

How the case is made and by whom are important. Allies are needed. The idea should be supported by the hospital clinicians and health workers who will be affected. The local medical committee's (LMC) support is essential. Patient opinion should be mobilized, from an epilepsy association, particularly a local patient group if this exists, and the Community Health Council. How the case is made will depend upon local circumstances, e.g. via the LMC or a commissioning forum, or directly to the Chief Executive of the Health Authority or Commission.

To assist in preparing a case, the main health needs and potential health gain for an average health authority of 500 000 are shown below.

Health needs for those with epilepsy in a population of 500 000

The numbers of patients and age/sex distribution given are based on an audit of 26 Doncaster practices and differ slightly from those in the documents referred to above.

Incidence and prevalence

Incidence is about 50–70 per 100 000, or **250–300 new cases each year** for this population. About double that number will be referred to hospital services (to general paediatrics and general medicine in the absence of neurology services). The incidence is highest in children and the elderly, with about 25% of new cases in those over 60 years old.

Prevalence is between five and seven per 1000, **about 2800 in total**. Figure 10.1 shows the age/sex distribution, which is fairly evenly distributed throughout late childhood and adult life. Those affected face education, employment and social problems. The severity of the condition varies. Thirty-five per cent (**700–1000**) will have more than one seizure each

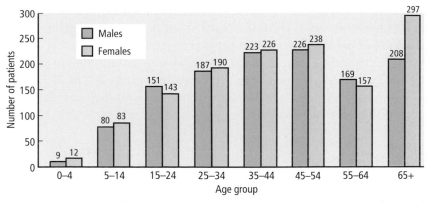

Fig. 10.1 Projected age/sex distribution of people with epilepsy in a population of 500 000. Based on an age/sex distribution from an audit carried out by Doncaster MAAG in 26 practices (*n* = 2599) and extrapolated to all practices in Doncaster (52). Prevalence in whole population equates to 5.2 per 1000.

month, 25% less than one seizure each month and about 40% will be fully controlled. A proportion will have associated neurological problems such as severe learning disability.

Mortality

Mortality rates are difficult to obtain, since deaths are normally attributed to other causes, e.g. underlying causes or a consequence such as drowning. Prospective surveys suggest that excess mortality is two to four times that of the population without epilepsy, and is greatest in children and young adults. Projections from a population survey in Nova Scotia [44] in which deaths as a result of seizures were found to be 2.68 per 100 000, suggest a mortality of **12–15 per annum**. Other excess deaths associated with epilepsy are an increased risk of suicide and deaths in young adults from the sudden unexplained death in epilepsy syndrome (SUDEP). Overall, there are likely to be **40–50 excess deaths annually as a result of epilepsy**.

Morbidity associated with epilepsy

Apart from the morbidity of simply experiencing seizures and associated neurological disabilities there are other effects: possibly as many as 10–25% [23] of those diagnosed as having epilepsy, **about 200–400, may not have epilepsy** but carry the label. Drug side-effects are a problem for most patients. Injuries associated with seizures are common, mainly minor injuries to the head, and include unnecessary damage to teeth by ignorant first-aiders. Projected figures indicate **150–170 injuries resulting from seizures per annum**.

The considerable psychosocial consequences to the individual and family and felt needs were fully discussed in Chapter 1. These include stigmatization, problems with education, employment, sport, and the need for information and counselling.

Potential for health gain in a population of 500 000

Some health gain lies in prevention. There is evidence that the incidence in children may be falling, perhaps due to improved maternity services, as well as demographic changes. The high incidence in the elderly (25%) total **60–75, is mainly associated with cerebrovascular disease/stroke**, some of which is potentially preventable. The other main preventable cause is head injury.

Most health gains stem from accurate diagnosis and optimum management, which require expertise and follow-up. Accurate diagnosis reduces the unnecessary misery of a diagnosis that has so many social consequences for some who do not have epilepsy (**approximately 200–400**) and ensures appropriate and effective treatment for those who do have it.

Optimum seizure control and education reduce the risk of seizure-related deaths (**12–15 per annum**) and accidents (**150–170 per annum**). Depression and suicide risk can be reduced by encouraging its recognition as a problem associated with epilepsy by doctors, and by the availability of liaison nurses on a telephone helpline.

There is a potential to reduce seizures and drug side-effects in about one-quarter of patients with epilepsy in the community [13]. Special epilepsy clinics have been found to be more effective in managing epilepsy than general neurology clinics [66]. Epilepsy services which in addition include specialist nurses are considered even more effective [24]. **Helping patients and families to cope, directly as well as by working with others such as teachers and employers, has emerged as being one of the most important achievements of epilepsy specialist nurses.**

Minimum 'critical mass' for an effective service

The evidence of health need may be overwhelming, as is the evidence for health gain, but most health districts have no specific services for epilepsy, and may have only a little to build on. As previously observed, recommendations for full services suggested in Appendix 3 are unlikely to be seen as realistic by many purchasers in the short term. The challenge is therefore to persuade purchasers to make a start, building upon whatever exists. There is, however, a minimum 'critical mass' for an effective service, which should include the following.

1 A specialist with an interest in epilepsy. Ideally a neurologist; if not, a physician who should be supported by links with a neurological centre.

2 Diagnostic services, EEGs, CT scan, magnetic resonance imaging (MRI), etc. (probably already being purchased).

3 A clinic for epilepsy at least monthly.

4 A Clinical Nurse Specialist in Epilepsy (CNSE), based in or with links to the community, including schools, employers, residential homes and offering open access (for the role of the nurse in epilepsy, see Chapter 11).

5 A clinical assistant/hospital practitioner.

6 Locally agreed objectives (Table 10.1), guidelines for shared care and policies for schools.

7 Training for doctors, nurses, care workers and teachers.

A district structure for epilepsy services

Ideally, patients with epilepsy and their relatives should have ready access to a level of expertise and advice which the severity or complexity of the condition indicates. Patients newly diagnosed or suspected of having epilepsy should be seen by an expert, usually within a few weeks, and those with chronic difficult epilepsy should have some specialist supervision. Since specialist neurologist services are scarce, we need to make effective

Table 10.1 Objectives for epilepsy management.

 1 To reduce preventable causes, e.g. cerebrovascular/stroke, head injury
 2 To secure early accurate diagnosis and classification of seizure type and if possible an epilepsy syndrome
 3 To identify any underlying cause
 4 To obtain optimum control with an appropriate anti-epileptic drug
 5 To avoid drug side-effects
 6 To identify those who might benefit from surgery
 7 To reduce deaths from preventable causes, e.g. seizure-related, suicide
 8 To assist patients and families to live life to the full by providing adequate counselling on the nature, dangers and consequences of epilepsy
 9 To assist and support children with epilepsy, parents and teachers with problems associated with education
 10 To assist and support patients and employers with problems associated with employment
 11 To provide information about supporting organizations

use of them. And we need speedy, reliable communications between doctors, liaison nurses and other health workers. As far as general practice is concerned, a GP with a special interest or expertise might undertake a major role in managing even difficult patients, but usually as many as 25–30% of patients will merit follow-up by a specialist service, which will involve some degree of shared care.

The structure in Table 10.2 is based upon guidelines used in Doncaster.

Table 10.2 A structure for care.

General practice care
1 Initial diagnosis
2 Patients with full control or infrequent seizures
3 Patients with variable control whom the GP feels competent to manage
4 Patients with poor control who appear not to be helped further by specialist services, or will not accept them

Hospital care
1 New patients—confirmation of diagnosis, identification of any underlying cause, recommendations regarding initial treatment, follow-up until control
2 Chronic, poorly controlled patients
3 Patients with relapse
4 Patients requiring specialist review, e.g. in pregnancy
5 Acute problems: status epilepticus, crescendo, clustering
6 Access to special centres for those with severe epilepsy, or other associated problems

Optional specialist review
1 To consider stopping treatment in remission
2 To consider newly available treatments, e.g. new drugs or surgery

Shared care
1 Almost all patients attending hospital will require shared care. Many require changes in drugs or dosage, and specialist epilepsy liaison nurses, where available, may prove crucial in facilitating this
2 Seizure diaries are essential for monitoring patients with frequent seizures. Co-operation cards and a management plan, preferably shared with the patient, greatly facilitate shared care

Liaison service (where available)
1 Provides a link in shared care with rapid access to the appropriate service
2 Provides supervision from clinic or general practice for changes in anti-epileptic therapy
3 Provides counselling and education, support in clinic and community with open access

Management in general practice

In the UK, the GP is seen as responsible for initial diagnosis and continuity of care. He or she is certainly usually the person best placed to get the evidence upon which an accurate diagnosis can be based, and whatever the extent of specialist services will be, to a greater or lesser extent, the person responsible for chronic long-term care.

It would be a sound basis for care if each practice had a policy or 'care plan' for its patients with epilepsy. This would specify how patients with new or chronic epilepsy would be looked after by the practice, and what would be expected from specialists. Will the practice expect specialists to provide continuing supervision of those with severe seizures? Having identified patients with continuing but infrequent seizures, will the practice intervene and optimize treatment or refer?

The respective roles of partners and practice nurses might be considered (Fig. 10.2; see also Chapter 11). Should one partner develop a special interest? (CSAG seem to think that this should happen; see Chapter 1) Review and counselling takes time and may need the restructuring of normal surgery appointments, sharing care with practice nurses or epilepsy specialist nurses. Some practices might consider setting up special epilepsy clinics, but the numbers may not be really sufficient to justify this except in a large practice, and patients might not like to attend something designated as an 'Epilepsy Clinic'. If it is to be done, some means of providing 'protected time'

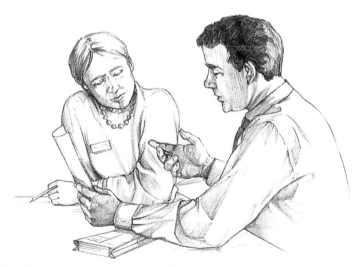

Fig. 10.2 GP discussing a patient with the practice nurse.

and payment along the lines of that for other chronic disease management will be desirable.

Knowing who the patients are is of course necessary, but a practice epilepsy register is constructed relatively easily from reviewing repeat prescribing, since most patients will be on anti-epileptic drugs (provided it is remembered that some anti-epileptic drugs are used for other reasons, e.g. carbamazepine for neuralgia).

The management of suspected new cases

Table 10.3 provides an outline for the management of suspected new cases of epilepsy. Suggestions for the initial work-up, diagnosis and early counselling have been described in detail earlier (Chapter 4, page 34). A major emphasis is on obtaining a witnessed description of events, before, during and after the 'attack'. If treatment has to be considered before a specialist opinion can be obtained, reference should be made to Chapter 5.

The management of existing cases

Table 10.4 outlines the management of existing patients with a diagnosis of epilepsy.

Table 10.3 Management in general practice: new cases (one or two per year per GP).

Secure an accurate diagnosis	A GP is in a key position to obtain and record detailed information about attacks soon after the events
Refer to specialist	For confirmation of the diagnosis Classification of seizure type Aetiology Possible syndrome classification Guidance on treatment
Initiate treatment	If seizures are frequent pending appointment and if confident about the diagnosis Information and counselling
Refer to Liaison Nurse/ Nurse	Counselling, support for carers and Practice families. The nurse may obtain details of attacks helpful to making the diagnosis, pending a specialist appointment
Refer to patient associations	For example, the British Epilepsy Association; see addresses of these on pages 167–168; also local support groups

Table 10.4 Management in general practice: existing cases.

Arrange regular review of patients on practice epilepsy register, depending on severity

Offer review to patients joining the practice with a diagnosis of epilepsy

Consider review of patients with frequent attendances at accident and emergency departments

At review, check:	The diagnosis: is it epilepsy? Seizure type?
	Seizure control (number of attacks, type of attack, seizure diary)
	Medication (appropriate? adequate?)
	Compliance
	Drug side-effects
	Serum levels (only if indicated)
	Co-operation card up to date
	Offer continued education/information about epilepsy
	Patient's changing circumstances, e.g. need to drive, contraception, pregnancy planning, employment. Agree plan and fix future review date
Consider intervention if:	Poor control: adjust medication—optimize and simplify if possible
	Change medication (with caution), preferably in liaison with a specialist (see page 59)
	If in prolonged remission, consider stopping medication (with caution), preferably in liaison with a specialist
Refer to specialist if:	Doubts about the diagnosis
	Poor seizure control
	Problems with medication
	Neurological deterioration
	For advice in changing circumstances, e.g. stopping treatment, pregnancy
	Consideration of new therapies, e.g. new drugs, surgery

Making a fresh and detailed review of every patient with epilepsy in a practice is obviously a demanding challenge and may take half an hour or more for each patient, particularly if descriptions of seizures are being sought from relatives. In the author's experience, much of the time is spent in answering the questions there was never an opportunity for those affected to ask before. The latter task is one which can be shared with a nurse, but whoever does it, Chapters 8 and 9 should help.

If at this point you are again wondering if you can possibly find the time, remember that there are only about 10–15 patients on the list of each GP, and that there is no doubt that patients really will benefit. Some of the arguments for review are set out in Chapter 5, page 57. How to set about a review is described in detail on page 58 and changing treatment on page 59.

The question of further training may possibly arise for both doctors and nurses. 'Neuroeducation' of York Health runs workshops up and down the country for GPs and practice nurses. Leeds Metropolitan University offers a professional diploma in epilepsy care as a distance learning package. The National Society for Epilepsy at the Chalfont Centre provides training for nurses in partnership with. Buckinghamshire Chilterns University College (see 'Sources of Help and Advice', Appendix 1).

Audit

Finally, after you have gone to the trouble to lobby for improved specialist services and improved the care provided in your practice, you might wish to audit your investment in time and energy. Appendix 2 comprises an audit pack which has now been used in over 400 practices. Its creators are happy for it to be used and would be interested to hear of your results.

The Role of the Nurse in Epilepsy 11

Without doubt, the arrival of the epilepsy specialist nurse on the scene in the late eighties has had a major impact on epilepsy services, and the subsequent expansion in numbers has been startling. Since the first post was established in Doncaster in 1988, there were at the last count 100 [11] or more epilepsy specialist nurses in post in the UK, including 39 Sapphire nurses funded by the BEA. The Epilepsy Specialist Nurse Association (ESNA) has 280 members, including 118 full members (employed exclusively in the field of epilepsy) and 165 associate members. The expansion has accompanied a long overdue increase in the number of epilepsy services in the UK, currently around 127 according to the CSAG report [11] and 100 (60 adult services and 40 children's services) according to the BEA. Recent reports [9–11] all stress the value of the specialist nurse in any epilepsy service. It may be that recognition of the potential contribution of nurse specialists has actually made the setting up of new services a realistic possibility. The specialist nurse, now known as 'Clinical Nurse Specialist in Epilepsy' (CNSE), has arrived and it is necessary to evaluate her or his effectiveness, and address the issues of training and role.

Nurses other than Clinical Nurse Specialists in Epilepsy are involved with epilepsy—learning disability nurses, some school nurses and nurses in primary care—and many of these are undertaking training in epilepsy.

Nurse training

Interest in training is impressive. The Leeds Metropolitan University 'Professional Diploma in Epilepsy Care', which is a distance learning package, has had an intake of over 350 in 4 years, with over 100 in the current year. Most students are nurses, from very differing backgrounds: hospital, community, primary care, a large group from learning disabilities, and a few school nurses. Buckinghamshire Chilterns University College, in partnership with the National Society for Epilepsy (NSE), provides part-time ENB courses (ENB N45) in a mixed mode of study blocks over 15 weeks. The NSE students are also from a variety of backgrounds. There are obviously many different roles in nursing associated with epilepsy care (see page 169 for details of courses).

The benefits

The benefits of having a specialist nurse with both a clinical and a liaison role in an epilepsy service were apparent almost immediately (see Chapter 10, pages 148–149), and subsequent reports have confirmed these findings [24]. In Doncaster, an audit [43] identified a reduced workload for GPs and consultants, fewer clinic visits for patients, increased support and counselling for patients and families, and significantly reduced levels of anxiety and depression.

Reports from the 'CARE' project in Cheshire [67,68] concluded that the Clinical Nurse Specialist in Epilepsy was 'a cost-effective cornerstone of a structured epilepsy service'. The 'CARE' project (Community Awareness and Resources for Epilepsy) is a partnership between a number of general practices and the David Lewis Centre. It carried out an assessment of epilepsy health needs, audited the use of health resources by the combined practice populations (30 000), established a model epilepsy service, and then audited the service. Among assessment findings, the diagnosis was considered incorrect in 23.8%. Results included a reduction in admissions to accident and emergency departments due to seizures from 16 to 5 per annum, hospital admissions from 16 to 3 per annum, and GP out-of-hours calls down from 18 to 1 per annum. There was evidence of improved seizure control, with 14% becoming seizure-free and almost a third reporting improvement. Initially, face-to-face review of all patients was by a consultant, but it was recognized that this was neither cost-effective nor sustainable, and the model that has evolved from the project is nurse-based.

One report on epilepsy specialist nurse-run clinics in primary care [69] found them to be well attended, a significant number of patients required drug changes and patients were better informed about their condition. Another report [70], from the patients' perspective, found that patients were less likely to report missing taking their anti-epileptic drugs, and it showed evidence of an improvement in communication and satisfaction, though not health status.

Overall, the Clinical Nurse Specialist in Epilepsy appears to have a major and developing role in improved epilepsy services.

Summary of benefits

- Improved compliance and fewer drug side-effects
- Improved seizure control and fewer injuries

- Support and counselling
- Improved knowledge and understanding of the condition
- Improved quality of life
- Less anxiety and depression
- Help with schools and employers
- Improved care during pregnancy, labour and postnatally
- Reduced emergency call-out for GPs
- Fewer hospital clinic and A&E visits
- Fewer emergency admissions

The role of the Clinical Nurse Specialist in Epilepsy

So what does the Clinical Nurse Specialist actually do? Responsibilities may range from the wide-ranging remit of the community-based nurse working in a district epilepsy service [24] to the nurse with more focused responsibilities, e.g. in a hospital clinic or department. Whatever the location, the nurse will share the care of the person with epilepsy with a multitude of professionals. These will include neurologists, paediatricians and other hospital staff, GPs, practice nurses, community nurses, midwives, clinical psychologists, social workers, community paediatricians and learning disability teams. There will be liaison with teachers, social services, housing departments, benefit advisers and employers.

The following list of objectives indicates the range of roles that *might* be met in a district service. Specialist nurses from different bases either in the community or clinic face the challenge of covering these roles in one way or another. Where a nurse is based will affect how this can be done, and it might be necessary to share roles between nurses in different bases. Whatever the arrangements, it is essential that the care of the person with epilepsy is co-ordinated, and it is here that the Nurse Specialist has a pivotal role.

The role of the Clinical Nurse Specialist in Epilepsy *may* include the following:
(The list is adapted from *Epilepsy Care—Making it Happen* [10])
- To operate an *open* referral system.
- To support and advise patients through the complicated process of starting, changing or withdrawing anti-epileptic medication.
- To investigate compliance issues—providing advice and pill wallets where appropriate and liaising with community pharmacists.
- To advise on other therapeutic approaches to epilepsy and simple measures to reduce seizures.
- To provide information, education and support to patients and families.

- To promote ownership and empowerment of patients with epilepsy.
- To establish self-help epilepsy groups.
- To act as a liaison between primary and secondary care.
- To provide information, education and support to the primary health care team.
- To undertake initial screening and review of all patients identified by practices with a primary diagnosis of epilepsy.
- To develop links with community pharmacists, local education authorities, social services, employers, disability employment advisers and housing departments.
- To develop links and teaching packages for local health providers, including: midwives, community learning disability services, community mental health services and student nurses.
- To attend clinical reviews of patients in learning disability community homes, community homes for the severely physically handicapped and those with autism.
- To attend case reviews in schools and for statementing of children.
- To set up a book/video library and resource centre.
- To set up a camcorder loan scheme to record seizure activity.
- To develop an epilepsy database of patients and participate in audit and research.

The list is quite awesome and few districts have anything approaching the range of activity implied, and some, as yet, lack the neurologist or other epilepsy specialist expertise to underpin a service. Where resources are limited, newly diagnosed cases and chronic cases in the specialist 'system' must take priority, and the review by the specialist nurse of long-established patients with the label of epilepsy in learning disability community homes, and in general practice, is less likely. This is a pity because there is ample evidence of the benefits of these activities [12,13,23,67,68], including: uncovering misdiagnosis, improving seizure control and reducing drug side-effects. However, there is undoubtedly a role for general practice and especially a practice nurse with epilepsy training, in reviewing epilepsy patients (see Chapter 10, page 157).

Where should the epilepsy specialist nurse work?

People generally find nurses more approachable and less threatening than they do doctors, and so confide more; this is so in any situation. A nurse who works solely in a clinic will achieve much because of this and other clinical skills, but visiting patients in their own homes adds an extra dimension. Patients in the security of their own homes, especially with someone they have already met, confide much more—and the homes themselves can tell a lot. Many of the problems, e.g. poor compliance, become clearer, and agreement on practical solutions can follow more readily.

Being able to visit nursing colleagues, GPs, schools, residential homes, etc. can be more effective than writing or telephoning, whether to discuss an individual patient's epilepsy management or ability to cope, or to discuss epilepsy issues and professional training.

It is desirable that an epilepsy specialist nurse, wherever based, can go out into the community.

What support is required?

Some things are obvious, but often there is a battle to get everything at once: an office, secretarial help, computers, telephone lines and answering machines; funds for pill wallets, literature, teaching resource materials, videos, camcorders to record fits; the list grows as a service grows. Some things, though, are vital: **ready access to an epilepsy specialist** associated with patients being managed; an agreed district protocol or set of guidelines to work within; individual patient management plans from the clinician responsible to guide and authorize clinical activities involving drug changes. Finally, professional isolation is to be avoided, and support from nursing colleagues both within the service, and possibly through ESNA, is desirable.

The role of the practice nurse

Inevitably, the role that a practice nurse will be able to fulfil will depend on the extent to which a practice and at least one partner are willing to structure epilepsy care. It will also depend upon having high quality, responsive local specialist epilepsy services, support from specialist nurses, and the nurse's own training. Some training might be provided locally by specialist nurses, but one of the courses suggested above for specialist nurses would be advisable if a significant role, such as that involving patient review, is intended.

The possibilities are considerable. Much of the suggested role for general practice outlined in Chapter 10, pages 155–158, can be undertaken by a practice nurse with suitable training and the support suggested above. It should involve home visiting where appropriate. It is unfortunate that epilepsy, despite the CSAG report [11], does not yet attract the NHS funding for chronic disease management that asthma and diabetes do. This makes funding nursing posts and service support such as books and leaflets a problem.

The role of the practice nurse *might* include the following tasks:

• To obtain a description about events before, during and after a suspected seizure from the individual and witnesses—crucial to making an accurate initial diagnosis or in reviewing the diagnosis.

• To provide counselling, information and support to patients and families.

• To encourage compliance—providing advice and pill wallets.

• To review existing patients, using a practice protocol, prior to case conferences with a GP and/or specialist nurse.

• To supervise care plans initiated by the GP or specialist—such as the complicated process of starting, changing or withdrawing medication.

• To act as a focal point within the practice for patients with epilepsy, their families and the practice team.

• To monitor adverse events—ensuring that patients who may have been admitted to an A&E department or presented with injuries following seizures are followed up.

• To liaise with specialist nurses, other practice nurses, community nurses, learning disability teams, schools and school nurses.

• To establish a practice epilepsy register and undertake an audit.

The role of the community learning disability nurse and the community learning disability epilepsy specialist nurse

(Adapted from East Yorkshire Community Healthcare NHS Trust role specification)

As people with learning disability in the UK have moved from large institutions into the community, their health needs are, on the whole, now met within primary care settings (see also Chapter 7, page 100). These needs can be considerable, and learning disability teams, including learning disability nurses, have evolved to meet many of these needs. Since 25–30% of people with learning disability also have epilepsy, often of a severe and difficult nature, an increasing number of nurses have taken training in epilepsy, and some services now employ nurses who specialize in both epilepsy and learning disability.

The learning disability nurse and epilepsy

The learning disability nurse, especially if a 'named nurse' for specific clients, is in a key position to gather information from clients, parents, carers, adult resource centres, respite homes and colleges to provide a comprehensive assessment (see Appendix 4). This would include information about:

- descriptions of seizures (including video recording);
- behavioural episodes;
- nature of learning disability;
- physical problems and limitations;
- medication, including side-effects and previous medication;
- recording of seizures;
- quality of life issues;
- results of previous investigations.

With suitable support and training, the learning disability nurse might also undertake many of the roles identified for the practice nurse (see above), e.g. sharing care plans with the epilepsy specialist nurse, GP or specialist, providing information, encouraging compliance and monitoring events (seizures and behaviour).

The learning disability epilepsy specialist nurse

The learning disability epilepsy specialist nurse would work closely with local epilepsy specialists and the clinical nurse specialists in epilepsy in the local epilepsy service. The epilepsy specialist nurse would co-ordinate care for the local population of people with a learning disability who also have epilepsy. Many of the roles might be very similar, or shared (see above for CNSE), but would include the following in particular:

- To determine the correct diagnosis of epilepsy.
- To determine the correct type of epilepsy.
- To ensure appropriate monitoring of seizure type, frequency and intensity.
- To ensure appropriate treatment, including correct use of drugs and complementary therapies.
- To improve clients' and carers' knowledge of epilepsy and its management.
- To promote patient's compliance with treatment.
- To set up a database of people with a learning disability for epidemiological research and audit purposes.
- To carry out an audit process to monitor outcomes.

Sources of Help and Advice

Epilepsy associations

British Epilepsy Association

Advice and Information Services, New Anstey House, Gate Way Drive, Yeadon, Leeds, LS19 7XY.
Telephone the Epilepsy Helpline on 0808 800 5050 (freephone) 9.00 am–4.30 pm Monday to Thursday and 9.00 am–4.00 pm on Fridays.
Website address: www.epilepsy.org.uk

The British Epilepsy Association helps people with epilepsy and their families by:
• Providing an advice and information service.
• Its Website and Online Community.
• Organizing talks, seminars and conferences and producing information pamphlets, videos and packs, and a newsletter *Epilepsy Today*.
• Supporting a national network of local self-help groups.
• Campaigning on behalf of people with epilepsy and acting as advocate for individuals facing problems with employment, benefits, legal and insurance matters.
• Combating negative attitudes and prejudice by improving understanding of epilepsy.
• Funding social research (non-laboratory).
Also at: BEA Northern Ireland Office, Graham House, Knockbrachen Healthcare Park, Belfast BT8 8BH, Tel: 028 9079 9076.

Epilepsy Association of Scotland

National Headquarters, 48 Govan Road, Glasgow G51 1JL, Tel: 0141 427 4911.
Helpline open between 1.00 pm and 4.30 pm weekdays, Tel: 0141 427 5225.

The Epilepsy Association of Scotland's activities and services include:
• Lobbying central government, local authorities and health boards on epilepsy matters.

- Promoting public awareness about epilepsy.
- Providing a telephone helpline.
- Maintaining an epilepsy resource centre—including a video library and a wide range of literature.
- Training a wide range of professional groups in understanding and managing epilepsy.
- Pursuing a vigorous appeals and marketing policy.
- Setting up and supporting local branches and groups.
- Providing a consultancy service.
- Providing community support for people with severe epilepsy.

The National Society for Epilepsy

Chalfont St Peter, Gerrards Cross, Buckinghamshire, Tel: 01494 601 300.
A source of advice, leaflets and videos.
Provides part-time courses in epilepsy for nurses in partnership with Buckinghamshire Chilterns University College. The (ENB N45) course, Nursing Care of the Individual with Epilepsy (30 credit points at level 2 or 3), is part-time in a mixed mode of study blocks over 15 weeks.

Mersey Region Epilepsy Association

Glaxo Neurological Centre, Norton Street, Liverpool L3 8LR, Tel: 0151 298 2666.

The Irish Epilepsy Association

249 Crumlin Road, Crumlin, Dublin 12, Tel: 00 3531 455 7500.

Epilepsy Wales

15 Chester Street, St Asaph, Denbighshire LL17 0RE, Tel: 01745 584 444.

Residential centres for people with epilepsy

Chalfont Centre for Epilepsy, Chalfont St Peter, Bucks SL9 0RJ, Tel: 01494 601 300.
David Lewis Centre, Warford, Alderley Edge, Cheshire SK0 7UD, Tel: 0156 564 0000.
Meath Home for Women and Girls with Epilepsy, Westbrook Road, Godalming, Surrey GU7 2QJ, Tel: 01483 415 095.

Parkhaven Trust, Liverpool Road South, Liverpool L31 8BR, Tel: 0151
526 4133.

Quarrier's, Quarrier's Village, Bridge of Weir, Renfrewshire PA11 3SD,
Tel: 01505 612 224.

St Elizabeth's School, Much Hadham, Herts SG10 6EW, Tel: 01279 843
451.

Schools for children with epilepsy

St Piers Lingfield, St Piers Lane, Lingfield, Surrey RH7 6PN, Tel: 01342
832 243.

St Elizabeth's School, Much Hadham, Herts SG10 6EW, Tel: 01279 843
451.

David Lewis Centre, Warford, Alderley Edge, Cheshire SK9 7UD, Tel:
0156 564 0000.

Assessment centres for epilepsy and epilepsy services

Department of Neurosciences, York District Hospital, Wigginton Road,
York YO3 7HE, Tel: 01904 631 313.

Chalfont Centre for Epilepsy, Chalfont St Peter, Bucks SL9 0RJ, Tel:
01494 601 300.

David Lewis Centre, Warford, Alderley Edge, Cheshire SK9 7UD, Tel:
0156 564 0000.

The Centre for Epilepsy, King's College Hospital, Mapother House, De
Crespigny Park, Camberwell, London SE5 8AS, Tel: 020 7277 1985.

Park Hospital for Children, Old Road, Headington, Oxford OX3 7LQ,
Tel: 01865 226 277.

National Hospital for Neurology and Neurosurgery, Queen Square, London
WC1N 3BG, Tel: 020 7837 3611.

The Walton Centre for Neurology and Neurosurgery, Lower Lane, Fazakerley,
Liverpool L9 7LJ, Tel: 0151 525 3611.

Department of Neuropsychiatry, Queen Elizabeth Psychiatric Hospital,
Mindelsohn Way, Edgbaston, Birmingham B15 2TH, Tel: 0121 678 2000.

Specialist nurse training

The National Society for Epilepsy (see address above) provides part-time
courses in epilepsy for nurses in partnership with Buckinghamshire
Chilterns University College. The (ENB N45) course, Nursing Care of the

Individual with Epilepsy (30 credit points at level 2 or 3), is part-time in a mixed mode of study blocks over 15 weeks.

Leeds Metropolitan University offers a Professional Diploma in Epilepsy Care. This is a distance learning package with an annual intake of 100. The diploma is split into three modules: clinical, social plus psychological, and the third in an area of study chosen by the student. Completion provides the diploma plus 45 CATS points at level 3. Applications to: The Course Administrator, Professional Diploma in Epilepsy Care, Centre for Community Neurological Studies, Faculty of Health and Environment, Leeds Metropolitan University, Calverley Street Leeds LS1 3BE.

Identification bracelets, etc.

Medic Alert Foundation, 1 Bridge Wharf, 156 Caledonian Road, London N1 9UU, Tel: 020 7833 3034.
SOS Talisman, 21 Grays Court, Ley St, Ilford, Essex, Tel: 020 8554 5579.
Tyser UK Ltd, Acorn House, Great Oaks, Basildon, Essex SS14 1AL, Tel: 01268 284 361.

Other useful addresses

Royal Society for the Prevention of Accidents, Rospa House, Edgbaston Park, 353 Bristol Road, Birmingham B5 7ST, Tel: 0121 248 2000.
Epilepsy Bereaved, PO Box 112, Wantage, Oxfordshire OX12 8XT, Tel: 01235 772 850.
Bereavement Contact line, Tel: 01235 772 852.

Disablement employment adviser

Contact your local Job Centre.

Driving licences

Medical Branch DVLA, Longview Road, Swansea SA99 1TU, Tel: 01792 783 750.

Books for adults

Chadwick, D. and Usiskin, S. *Living with Epilepsy*. London: Macdonald Optima, 1991.

Chappell, B. and Crawford, P. *Epilepsy at Your Fingertips*. London: Class Publishing, 1999.

Oxley, J. and Smith, J. *The Epilepsy Reference Book*. London: Faber & Faber, 1991.

Books for children

Appleton, R. *The Illustrated Junior Encyclopaedia of Epilepsy*. Roby Education, 1995. Age range: 7 years upwards (good for adults too).

Appleton, R. *Hand in Hand*. Marion Merrell Dow, 1993. Age range: 7–14 years.

Llewellyn, K. *My Mum has Epilepsy*. Karen Llewellyn, 1994. Age range: 5–9 years.

Videos

Parents' and Young Children's Information Pack.

Parents' and Young Adults' Information Pack.

All books and videos available from the British Epilepsy Association.

2 Managing Epilepsy in General Practice: Audit*

Why audit?

- Because audit activity is expected.
- It can lead to improved patient care.
- It can be thought-provoking and interesting.

Why epilepsy?

- It is common, without being too common, so the audit should not take too long.
- People with epilepsy in the practice are easy to identify.
- Previous studies have shown that there is potential for improvement in the management of epilepsy.
- Any improvement is often manageable without an excessive time commitment.

Strategy

Whilst it is a good idea for one member of the practice to promote the audit, it is important that all GPs and staff become involved. Involvement of all members of the team in this discussion may generate enthusiasm and commitment to the project.

Step 1: preparing for the audit

Arrange a meeting of all the partners. Consider inviting practice nurses and office staff, especially if they are going to do some of the work collecting information.

* Prepared by Bill Hall, General Practitioner, Settle, N. Yorks, and Brian Chappell, Neuroeducation. Correspondence to: Neuroeducation, PO Box 17, Golcar, Huddersfield HD7 4YX.

The purpose of the meeting is to consider what your practice thinks the standards of care for your patients with epilepsy should be.

Possible discussion points may include some of the following.
• Should all patients suspected of having epilepsy be referred to a consultant for investigation?
• Should patients be regularly followed up by a hospital consultant?
• What are the aims of treatment? Should patients be completely free of seizures? Should patients have a say in their treatment?
• Which anti-epileptic drugs would you consider to be first-line treatments?
• How often should drug levels be monitored? Are they more important than seizure control?
• When should polytherapy be considered? Is it ever necessary?
• How often should patients with epilepsy be seen by their GP?
• What information should be recorded in the notes? Should recording the number of seizures in the last year be an aim?
• What information (e.g. careers advice) should patients with epilepsy be given and who should give it?

If you are interested, more information on these topics can be supplied.

Someone needs to record what the practice consensus is on these discussion points, then– hey presto!—you have your practice's own standards of care for your patients with epilepsy.

Step 2: collecting the information

1 A member of staff (this could be a GP, a receptionist, practice nurse or secretary) should scrutinize the repeat prescriptions for 3 months and keep a list of patients who are on anti-epileptic drugs (see 'Drug list', below). You can expect between 5 and 15 for an average GP's list.

Alternative methods might be to use your computer, if you have one. Remember, some GPs may issue repeat prescriptions on home visits, and some patients may get their drugs from hospital. If you can remember who these patients are, that is fine; if not, it does not matter too much. This should identify all the patients who have epilepsy in the practice except:
  (a) those who are non-compliant; and
  (b) those who have a history of epilepsy, but are no longer being treated.
2 Obtain notes (by receptionist?) for all identified patients.
3 Scrutinize notes to see why these patients are taking anti-epileptics. (Doctor, practice nurse, trainee?) Discard patients who do not have a history of epilepsy. Some will be taking anti-epileptics for pain relief, depression

or glaucoma. *Note.* There may be quite a few, and it may be difficult to make clear decisions.

4 Collect information (by doctor?) required to complete the sample grid below. The following pieces of information outlined below may be useful, but you will possibly be interested in other topics. Remember that each additional item searched for increases the time taken.

This job is the most time-consuming. Depending on the state of your records, allow 10 minutes per set of notes, i.e. 1–2.5 hours per GP.

Suggested areas of information to collect

- Practice list size?
- Number of patients identified with epilepsy?
- Age of the patients?
- Sex of the patients?
- Number of drugs each patient is taking?
- Which drug(s) each patient is taking? (use the Drug List below, and codes)
- Does the repeat prescription match the notes?
- Number of seizures each patient has had in the last year?
- When was each patient last seen for any reason?
- When was each patient last seen about his/her epilepsy?
- When did each patient last visit a hospital consultant about his/her epilepsy?
- Has written information about epilepsy and its management been provided and recorded in the notes?
- Your additions, if required.

Step 3: making sense of the information

How you approach this section will very much depend on your areas of priority decided at Step 1.

The following suggestions may help to clarify your thoughts for assessing the data, but feel free to add any of your identified areas.

- How many patients in each age band: 0–10, 11–20, 21–30, etc.?
- How many males/females?
- Average number of anti-epileptic drugs per patient?
- Percentage of each anti-epileptic drug used as a proportion of total usage of all anti-epileptic drugs?
- Number of seizures per patient per annum? 0, 1–6, 7–12, 13–24, over 24 ('not recorded' likely to be most common).

- Patient last seen; any reason? Last month, 1–3 months, 4–6 months, 7–12 months, over 12 months.
- Patient last seen for epilepsy? Categories as previous question.
- Last hospital consultant visit? Categories as previous two questions.
- Record of information on epilepsy given? Percentage yes/no.

Step 4: discussing what you have discovered

The practice team needs to reconvene to discuss the findings. It helps if someone records the practice's conclusions.
- Present results.
- Discuss the implications.
- Plan the future management of patients with epilepsy—you may want to make some changes.
- Decide on a time for the next audit—it is a good idea to repeat the exercise to see if you have improved patient care.

Drug list

Code	Drug name
1	carbamazepine (Tegretol, Tegretol Retard)
2	sodium valproate (Epilim, Epilim Chrono)
3	phenytoin (Epanutin)
4	ethosuximide (Zarontin, Emeside)
5	vigabatrin (Sabril)
6	clobazam (Frisium)
7	clonazepam (Rivotril)
8	phenobarbitone (Luminal, Prominal)
9	primidone (Mysoline)
10	acetazolamide (Diamox)
11	lamotrigine (Lamictal)
12	gabapentin (Neurontin)
13	valproic acid (Convulex)
14	topiramate (Topamax)
15	tiagabine (Gabitril)
16	oxcarbazepine (Trileptal)

NAME OF PRACTICE

PRACTICE LIST SIZE

TOTAL PATIENTS WITH EPILEPSY ON THIS SHEET																			
Initials of patients																			
Actual age																			
Sex (M or F)																			
Number of drugs for epilepsy																			
Which drugs (see code)																			
Prescription matches notes																			
Number of seizures last year (NR–not recorded, or actual number)																			
Patient last seen, any reason																			
Patient last seen, epilepsy																			
Last hospital consultant visit (NR–not recorded)																			
Info on epilepsy given (NR–not recorded)																			

Purchasing and Providing Epilepsy Outpatient Services: A Guide to Good Practice*

Does your district currently provide the following epilepsy services?

• Access to a local dedicated epilepsy clinic.
• Readily available and easily understood information about specific types of epilepsy and seizures and any consequential investigations.
• Easy access to a specialist interdisciplinary team including:
   (a) a neurologist or other specialist provider with training expertise and an interest in managing newly diagnosed epilepsy;
   (b) a non-medical specialist trained in epilepsy and communication skills, e.g. epilepsy specialist (liaison) nurse;
   (c) social worker;
   (d) occupational therapist.
• Access to local magnetic resonance imaging (MRI) or computed tomography (CT) scanner.
• Access to an epilepsy helpline and readily available contact with voluntary organizations.
• Access to a paediatric neurologist specializing in epilepsy with a waiting time of no longer than 4 weeks.
• Access to a neurosciences centre with a waiting time of no longer than 4 weeks.
• Access to counselling services, including preconceptual counselling for women.

---

* By the Epilepsy Task Force and the Joint Epilepsy Council, published in 1995. The Epilepsy Task Force is an action-led initiative designed to address current shortfalls in care. The Epilepsy Task Force representatives are drawn from a range of professional and consumer bodies involved in epilepsy care, including neurologists, neuropsychiatrists, paediatric neurologists, GPs, Family Health Service Authority medical advisers, support groups and people with epilepsy.

The Joint Epilepsy Council (JEC) is a consortium of voluntary organizations and specialist centres involved in caring for people with epilepsy in the UK and Ireland. **177**

• A clear policy in relation to extracontractual referrals and the right to refer to a specialist centre.

Purchasing these services will lead to the provision of a good epilepsy service. Further information is provided below.

Introduction

This document seeks to establish the principle of purchasing outpatient epilepsy services. It aims to provide minimum standards of care and focuses on secondary care provision.

It is common for epilepsy services to be purchased under 'general neurology services'. Experience with dedicated epilepsy services has shown health gain benefits, and purchasers are encouraged to consider distinguishing epilepsy services within their purchasing specification. This will not necessarily involve the allocation of extra resources and will facilitate effective purchasing.

The following information may be useful to benchmark clinical services.

Epilepsy is the most common serious neurological disorder. In a UK health district population of 250 000, there are approximately 2000 patients with epilepsy. Six hundred of these will either experience frequent seizures or suffer unacceptable drug-related side-effects and will disproportionately consume health service resources. There is abundant evidence that the current service is inadequate and that potential for significant health gain is being lost [1,2]. A close working relationship between hospital and primary health care teams is therefore a major consideration.

Purchasers should grasp the opportunity to develop shared care protocols between hospital and family practitioner services, and to move towards 'one stop' clinics where initial assessment, consultation and investigations are conducted during a single visit.

In this way, diagnosis and appropriate shared care treatment can be agreed immediately. The development of epilepsy liaison posts, such as epilepsy liaison officers from professions allied to medicine, would greatly assist this process. Indeed, the Epilepsy Specialist Nurses Association (ESNA) is already in a position to set the necessary standards [3]. Such developments are likely to contribute to realistic target setting in the medium-term future, and will be addressed in more detail in future editions of this framework.

There are additional considerations.

1 Any framework for epilepsy care should separate the needs of adults from those of children and young people. Purchasers should be able to make the necessary distinction and adjust their policies accordingly.

2 People with seizure disorders often present at accident and emergency departments. Purchasers and providers should establish a clear policy of how these people's problems are managed, in particular establishing a liaison between family practitioners and specialist services for follow-up.

New patient referrals

Adults

Numbers

About 500 adults per year in a UK health district population of 250 000 may present to the primary health care team service with fits, faints or funny turns. Referral on to hospital opinion is likely to be requested in at least 250 of these.

Outpatient waiting list time

Epileptic phenomena are distressing and alarming to patients, and may occasionally represent medical conditions with a serious prognosis. Consequently, there should not be undue delay in seeing new referrals by the hospital service. It is therefore recommended that a maximum waiting time by the hospital service for a new outpatient appointment should be no longer than 4 weeks.

Children and young people

The number initially presenting are similar to adults, i.e. referral from primary health care to hospital with possible epilepsy is likely to be at least 250 patients per 250 000 population per year, and new outpatient appointments should be offered within 4 weeks of referral.

Initial investigation and management

Adults

Manpower

Patients with a potential diagnosis of epilepsy should be seen initially by a physician with expertise and interest in the subject. This consultation would ideally be part of a general neurology service, in which the level of epilepsy services provision was specified, and in which there was a neurologist with special responsibility for the epilepsy service.

With the present shortage of neurologists, there is the option in some areas of the country separately to purchase an epilepsy service from other specialist providers, e.g. neuropsychiatry or clinical pharmacology, provided that the physician concerned has training, expertise and an interest in managing newly diagnosed epilepsy.

Whoever is leading, there are other staff who should be part of the initial diagnosis team. This must include a non-medical specialist trained in epilepsy and communication skills, for example, an epilepsy specialist (liaison) nurse, social worker, occupational therapist, or any of a number of other professionals.

It is also essential that there should be access to counselling services, information provision and contact with voluntary organizations. These aspects require close co-operation between hospital and primary care, and how they are achieved locally should be part of each service specification.

Initial investigations

Investigations at this stage will include electroencephalogram (EEG) recording (315 recordings per year for this population) and neuroimaging. Up to 200 computed tomography (CT) scans are likely to be required per year as part of the screening process. The imaging investigation of choice for localization-related epilepsy is magnetic resonance (MR) scanning. In this population, a further 45 MR scans per year should be requested in adults. Serum anticonvulsant monitoring is unlikely to exceed 500 requests per year in this initially presenting group.

Appointments and numbers

The following figures refer to physician contact and do not include time that should be spent with appropriate non-medical specialists. The first appointment is likely to take 30 minutes with the physician. All patients are most likely to return for at least one further visit, for which at least 15 minutes should be allowed, to discuss results of investigations. By this time, a provisional diagnosis of epilepsy will have been made in about 105 patients and treatment commenced, and the other 120 will have been referred back to the GP or on to other services. After no more than two further appointments of 15 minutes each, some 15 more patients will be diagnosed as not having epilepsy, while 53 of the remaining 90 will enter early remission with treatment. This should leave no more than 37 for continuing follow-up.

In order to comply with patient charter standards, urgent action is required to identify medical epilepsy specialists.

Children and young people

Manpower

Children and young people with a potential diagnosis of epilepsy should be seen initially by a physician with expertise and an interest in the subject. This consultation is likely to be part of a general paediatric service, in which the level of epilepsy services provision is specified, and in which there is a paediatrician with special responsibility for the epilepsy service.

Other staff who should be part of the initial diagnosis team must include a non-medical specialist trained in epilepsy and communication skills, for example, an epilepsy specialist (liaison) nurse, occupational therapist, or any of a number of other professionals.

It is also essential that there should be access to counselling services, information provision and contact with voluntary organizations. It is important to recognize the need for families to talk to others for mutual support.

Children with epilepsy often underachieve at school and there may be special educational issues to address. The presence in the team of an appropriately trained psychologist is recommended, who would ensure a link between child health services and education services.

Initial investigations

Investigations at this stage will include EEG (315 recordings per year for this population) and neuroimaging. Up to 200 CT scans are likely to be required per year as part of the screening process. The imaging investigation of choice for localization-related epilepsy is MR scanning. In this population, a further 45 MR scans per year should be requested in children. Serum anticonvulsant monitoring is unlikely to exceed 500 requests per year in this population. Metabolic screening will be required in approximately 50 cases.

Appointments and numbers

The following figures refer to physician contact and do not include time that should be spent with the appropriate non-medical specialist. The first appointment is likely to take 45 minutes with the paediatrician or paediatric neurologist. All children and young people and their parents are most likely to return for at least one further visit, for which 30 minutes should be allowed, to discuss results of investigations. By this time, a provisional diagnosis of epilepsy will been made in about 105 and treatment commenced, and the other 120 will have been referred back to the primary health care team or on to other services. After no more than two further appointments of 15 minutes each, some 15 more will be diagnosed as not having epilepsy. It is customary for the remaining 90 to remain in touch with paediatric services. Some 53 will enter early remission with treatment, requiring fewer follow-up appointments, while the remaining 37 will be seen more often.

Follow-up

Adults

Approximately 250 adults will be attending the epilepsy clinic besides the newly diagnosed group. These will include patients with refractory epilepsy having ongoing follow-up and patients re-referred by the family practitioner for various reasons including recurrence or worsening of seizures, advice regarding tailing off medication after prolonged remission, preconceptual counselling, or the management of epilepsy in pregnancy. Such a group will each require an average of four 15-minute appointments per year. Also, patients and their family practitioners need to be able to contact the epilepsy service between appointments for telephone advice, or to bring an appointment forward in an emergency. An extra 50 appointments per year should be allowed for this.

Where seizures are continuing 2 years after initiation of treatment, or where there are psychiatric complications, referral on to an 'epilepsy plus' service for assessment and, where appropriate, pre-surgical evaluation is recommended. These may account for up to 20 referrals onward per year in this population. A further 500 serum drug levels per year may be requested in this group.

Children and young people

Approximately 500 children and young people will be attending the epilepsy clinic beside the newly diagnosed group. At least half of these will be in remission with treatment and require no more than two 15-minute appointments per year. The remainder may need an average of four appointments per year.

Parents and GPs need to be able to contact the epilepsy service between appointments for telephone advice, or to bring an appointment forward in an emergency. An extra 50 appointments per year should be allowed for this. A further 500 serum drug levels per year may be requested in this group.

Chronic epilepsy: epilepsy plus service

This should be provided at the level of a neurosciences centre, with each centre covering a population of approximately 2.5 million. Thus, a typical region is likely to have at least two centres located in areas of high population. The components and activities of this service are described in the Epilepsy Needs Document [1] and may include a special assessment unit. Of the 20 adults and 20 children per year who may be referred on from each district level, surgery may be offered in 10 (rendering eight seizure-free or greatly remitted), and non-epileptic seizures will be diagnosed and treated in 15. The remaining 15 may be referred back to the district service. The district service should be aware of such options as special educational provision and adult residential care.

Audit

Epilepsy is a highly suitable topic for outpatient service audit. Appropriate process measures (with suggested targets in brackets) include the following.
- Time to first appointment (less than 4 weeks).
- Waiting time for relevant investigations (less than 4 weeks for EEG, scans).
- Percentage of patients who undergo investigation by scanning (50%).
- Percentage of patients seizure-free 2 years from initial diagnosis (70%).
- Percentage of patients taking more than one anti-epileptic drug (< 30%).
- Percentage of patients discharged to GP in 1 year (80% all adult and 50% all child referrals).
- Percentage of patients in whom a 'counselling checklist' has been completed, including:
    (a) preconceptual counselling (100% women of childbearing age);
    (b) advice about driving regulations (100% over 17 years);
    (c) employment (100% under 65 years);
    (d) contact with voluntary organizations (100%).

• Rate of referral to 'epilepsy plus' services (20 adults and 20 children per year per 250 000 population).

An example package for auditing a hospital epilepsy service has been developed by the Research Unit of the Royal College of Physicians [4].

Totals

Adults

	Patients × time	Hours
New patient appointments per year	250 at 30 minutes*	125
First follow-up	250 at 15 minutes*	62.5
Second follow-up	105 at 15 minutes	26.25
Third follow-up	105 at 15 minutes	26.25
Total follow-ups beyond first year	1000 at 15 minutes	250
Brought-forward appointments	50 at 15 minutes	12.5

* These must be regarded as absolute minimum figures. Where the service carries a teaching commitment, 50% extra should be allowed. Many epilepsy specialists consider at least 1 hour to be appropriate for the first appointment, and 30 minutes for the second. Such a level of service should be at least a medium- to long-term aim. However, in the mid-1990s the immediate application of such a standard will result in demand rapidly outstripping supply. Therefore, the above figures are given because they should be reasonably achievable in 1995–96 in all parts of the UK. Once the principle of purchasing epilepsy services is established, quality assurance and audit procedures should demonstrate the need for future investment, training and service improvement.

The total = 502.5 hours per year medical contact plus one full-time equivalent non-medical specialist(s) trained in epilepsy and communication skills, for example, an epilepsy specialist nurse, counsellor, social worker or occupational therapist.

	Hours
EEGs per year	315
CT scans per year	200
MR scans per year	45
Serum drug levels per year (new presentations)	500
Serum drug levels per year (follow-ups)	500

Children

	Patients × time	Hours
New patient appointments per year	250 at 45 minutes*	187.5
First follow-up	250 at 30 minutes*	125
Second follow-up	105 at 15 minutes	26.25
Third follow-up	105 at 15 minutes	26.25
Total follow-ups beyond first year	2000 at 15 minutes	500
Telephone contact in emergency	100 at 15 minutes	25
Brought-forward appointments	50 at 15 minutes	12.5

*See the note above under adult services regarding timing of new patient appointment and first follow-up. The figures for children also represent absolute minimum requirements. Longer initial appointment times need to be allowed than in adult services because of the involvement of the family.

The total = 902.5 hours per year medical contact plus one full-time equivalent non-medical specialist(s) trained in epilepsy and communication skills, and a half full-time equivalent psychologist.

	Hours
EEGs per year	315
CT scans per year	200
MR scans per year	45
Serum drug levels per year (new presentations)	500
Serum drug levels per year (follow-ups)	500
Metabolic screening per year	50

References

1 Brown, S., Betts, T., Chadwick, D., Hall, W., Shorvon, S. and Wallace, S. An Epilepsy Needs Document. *Seizure* 1993; 2: 91–103.
2 Taylor, M.P., Readman, S., Hague, B., Boulter, V., Hughes, L. and Howell, S. A district epilepsy service, with community-based specialist liaison nurses and guidelines for shared care. *Seizure* 1994; 3: 121–127.
3 The Epilepsy Specialist Nurses Association (secretary Sister L. Lawton, c/o The David Lewis Centre, Mill Lane, Warford, near Alderley Edge, Cheshire SK9 7UD).
4 Royal College of Physicians. *Audit Protocol for Case Notes of a Patient with Newly Diagnosed Epilepsy*, 1992. Further details from: Research Unit, Royal College of Physicians, 11 St Andrews Place, Regents Park, London NW1 4LE.

4 Community Nurse Learning Disability Assessment of Epilepsy

This assessment instrument is supported by guidelines which are similar to material in this book. Copies of the 'guidelines' and the assessment pack can be obtained from: Heather Gregory, Community Nurse Learning Disability, The Grovehill Outreach Centre, Beckview Road, Beverley, East Yorkshire.

Hull and East Riding Community Health NHS Trust

COMMUNITY NURSE LEARNING DISABILITY ASSESSMENT OF EPILEPSY

SECTION 1 – CLIENT DETAILS

Name.. DoB...... /........./ .....

Address ....

Name of Community Nurse... Base ....

GP details ....

Consultant name and clinical details ....

SECTION 2 – SEIZURE DETAILS

Cause of epilepsy? *(if known)* ....

Other disabilities or health-related problems? *(if known)*...................................

Does the client have more than one type of seizure?   YES ☐   NO ☐

1   Description *(see guidelines)*...

....

....

....

....

International League Against Epilepsy Classification ,...

Age at onset of epilepsy........................ Diagnosis of seizure based on ....

Frequency of seizures........................... Date of last seizure ..../........ /..........

If other seizure type please complete

2   Description *(see guidelines)*...

....

....

....

....

International League Against Epilepsy Classification ....

Age at onset of epilepsy........................ Diagnosis of seizure based on ....

Frequency of seizures........................... Date of last seizure ..../........ /..........

Pseudo-seizures?   YES ☐   NO ☐
Description *(see guidelines)*..
....

Does the client present with any unsettled behaviour?   YES ☐   NO ☐
Description *(see guidelines)*..
....
....

SECTION 3 – QUALITY OF LIFE ISSUES

Social life/skills *(see guidelines)*..
....
....

Transport *(see guidelines)*...
....
....

Day Care/Employment/Education *(see guidelines)*.................................
....
....

Medication *(see guidelines)*...
....
....

Respite care *(see guidelines)*..
....
....

Contraception *(see guidelines)*...
....
....
....

Sleep patterns *(see guidelines)*..
....
....
....

SECTION 4 – RECORDING OF SEIZURES

How and where are the seizures recorded? ....

Are all key people aware of recording seizures?　YES　☐　NO　☐

Is the method of recording portable?　　　　　YES　☐　NO　☐

Does the record include:

	YES	NO		YES	NO
Clear definition	☐	☐	Medication changes	☐	☐
All seizure types	☐	☐	Treatment responses	☐	☐
Who completes the record	☐	☐	Triggers	☐	☐

SECTION 5 – INVESTIGATION RESULTS

EEG　　　　　　　　　　Date　　　　　　　Place

If more than 3　　　1　　......./ ..../ ....　　....................................

put first, last and　　2　　......./ ..../ ....　　....................................

one other　　　　　　3　　......./ ..../ ....　　....................................

Summary of results ....

....

AMBULATORY EEG　　　　Date　　　　　　　Place

　　　　　　　　　　　　1　　......./ ..../ ....　　....................................

　　　　　　　　　　　　2　　......./ ..../ ....　　....................................

Summary of results ....

CT SCAN　　　　　　　　Date　　　　　　　Place

　　　　　　　　　　　　1　　......./ ..../ ....　　....................................

　　　　　　　　　　　　2　　......./ ..../ ....　　....................................

Summary of results ....

....

MRI SCAN　　　　　　　　Date　　　　　　　Place

　　　　　　　　　　　　1　　......./ ..../ ....　　....................................

　　　　　　　　　　　　2　　......./ ..../ ....　　....................................

Summary of results ....

....

PHYSICAL EXAMINATIONS

....

....

OTHER SPECIALIST INVESTIGATIONS

....

SECTION 6 – MEDICATION

Name of current medication   Dosage   Date medication started

..../............./.........
..../............./.........
..../............./.........
..../............./.........
..../............./.........
..../............./.........

How often is medication reviewed? ....   Date of last review ...../..../....

Medication reviewed by ....

Any known side-effects...
....

Has blood monitoring been undertaken?   YES   ☐   NO   ☐

If YES please state when ..../........./.......   Results ....

Previous medication

Name of medication	Dosage (if known)	Date discontinued	Reason discontinued
....	....	....	....
....	....	....	....
....	....	....	....
....	....	....	....

SECTION 7 – OUTCOME OF ASSESSMENT AND ACTION TAKEN

SEIZURE DETAILS

....
....
....
....
....

QUALITY OF LIFE ISSUES

....
....
....
....
....

RECORDING OF SEIZURE DETAILS

....
....
....
....
....

INVESTIGATION RESULTS

....
....
....
....
....

MEDICATION

....
....
....
....
....

PLEASE COMPLETE, REFERRING TO GUIDELINES

DATE	TIME	BEFORE THE SEIZURE	WHAT HAPPENED	HOW LONG DID THE SEIZURE LAST?	AFTER THE SEIZURE/RECOVERY	RECOVERY TIME

Document Date March 2000
Review Date March 2001

References and Recommended Further Reading

References

1 Taylor, J. (ed.) *Selected Writings of John Hughlings Jackson*, Vol. 1: *On Epilepsy and Epileptiform Convulsions*. London: Hodder and Stoughton, 1931. Reprinted 1958 by Basic Books, New York.

2 Central Health Services Council. *Report of the Subcommittee on the Medical care of Epileptics*. London: HMSO, 1956.

3 Central Health Services Council. *People with Epilepsy*. London: HMSO, 1969.

4 Morgan, J.D. and Kurtz, Z. *Special Services for People with Epilepsy in the 1970s*. London: HMSO, 1987.

5 Department of Health and Social Security. *Report of the Working Group on Services for People with Epilepsy*. London: HMSO, 1986.

6 Duncan, J.S. and Hart, Y.M. Medical services. In: Laidlaw, J., Richens, A. and Chadwick, D. (eds). *A Textbook of Epilepsy*. Edinburgh: Churchill Livingstone, 1993: 705–722.

7 Brown, S., Betts, T., Chadwick, D., Hall, W., Shorvon, S. and Wallace, S. An Epilepsy Needs Document. *Seizure* 1993; 2: 91–103.

8 Brown, S., Betts, T., Crawford, P., Hall, B., Shorvon, S. and Wallace, S. Epilepsy needs revisited: a revised epilepsy needs document for the UK. *Seizure* 1998; 7: 435–446.

9 Epilepsy Task Force. *Epilepsy Task Force Service Development Kit*. London: Epilepsy Task Force, 1999.

10 Epilepsy Advisory Board. *Epilepsy Care—Making it Happen: A toolkit for today*. Leeds: British Epilepsy Association, 1999.

11 Clinical Standards Advisory Group. *Services for Patients with Epilepsy*. London: HMSO, 1999.

12 Taylor, M.P. A job half done. *J R Coll Gen Pract* 1980; 30: 456–465.

13 Taylor, M.P. Epilepsy in a Doncaster practice: audit and change over eight years. *J R Coll Gen Pract* 1987; 37: 116–119.

14 Shorvon, S.D., Chadwick, D., Galbraith, A.W. and Reynolds, E.H. One drug for epilepsy. *Br Med J* 1978; 1: 474–476.

15 Shorvon, S.D. and Reynolds, E.H. Reduction in polypharmacy for epilepsy. *Br Med J* 1979; 2: 1023–1025.

16 Lloyd Jones, A. Medical audit of the care of patients with epilepsy in one group practice. *J R Coll Gen Pract* 1980; 30: 396–400.

17 Goodman, I. Auditing care of epilepsy in a group practice. *Practitioner* 1983; 227: 435–436.

18 McCluggage, J.R., Ramsey, H.C., Irwin, W.G. and Dowds, M.F. Anticonvulsant therapy in a general practice population in Northern Ireland. *J R Coll Gen Pract* 1984; 34: 24–31.

19 Cooper, G.L. and Huitson, A. An audit of the management of patients with epilepsy in thirty practices. *J R Coll Gen Pract* 1986; 36: 204–208.

20 Hall, W.W. and Ross, D. General practice study of the care of epileptic patients. *Practitioner* 1986; 230: 661–665.

21 Presley, P. An audit of epilepsy in general practice. *Practitioner* 1989; 233: 1009–1014.

22 Smith, D., Defalla, B.A. and Chadwick. D.W. The misdiagnosis of epilepsy and the management of refractory epilepsy in a specialist clinic *Q J Med* 1999; 92: 15–23.

23 Scheepers B., Clough P. and Pickles, C. Misdiagnosis of epilepsy: results of a population study. *Seizure* 1998; 7, 403–406.

24 Taylor, M.P., Readman, S., Hague, B., Boulter, V., Hughes, L. and Howell, S. A district epilepsy service, with community-based specialist liaison nurses and guidelines for shared care. *Seizure* 1994; 3: 121–127.

25 Crombie, D., Cross, K., Fry, J. *et al.* A survey of the epilepsies in general practice. *Br Med J* 1960; 2: 416–422.

26 Pond, D., Bidwell, B. and Stein, L. A survey of 14 general practices. 1. Medical and demographic data. *Psychiatr Neurol Neurochir* 1960; 63: 641–644.

27 Sander, J.W.A.S., Hart, Y.M., Johnson, A.L. and Shorvon, S.D. National General Practice Study of Epilepsy: newly diagnosed epileptic seizures in a general population. *Lancet* 1990; 336: 1267–1274.

28 Hart, Y.M., Sander, J.W.A.S., Johnson, A.L. and Shorvon, S.D. National General Practice Study of Epilepsy: recurrence after first seizure. *Lancet* 1990; 336: 1271–1274.

29 Cockerell, O.C., Johnson, A.L., Sander, J.W.A.S., Hart, Y.M. and Shorvon, S.D. Remission of epilepsy: results from the National General Practice Study of Epilepsy. *Lancet* 1995; 346: 140–144.

30 Manford, M., Hart, Y.M., Sander, J.W.A.S. and Shorvon, S.D. National General Practice Study of Epilepsy: partial seizure patterns in a general population. *Neurology* 1992; 42: 1911–1917.

31 Manford, M., Hart, Y.M., Sander, J.W.A.S. and Shorvon, S.D. The National General Practice Study of Epilepsy. The syndromic classification of the International League Against Epilepsy applied to epilepsy in a general population. *Arch Neurol* 1992; 49: 801–808.

32 Chaplin, J.E., Lasso, R.Y., Shorvon, S.D. and Floyd, M. National General Practice Study of Epilepsy: the social and psychological effects of a recent diagnosis of epilepsy. *Br Med J* 1992; 304: 1416–1418.

33 Cockerell, O.C., Hart, Y.M., Sander, J.W.A.S. and Shorvon, S.D. The cost of epilepsy in the United Kingdom: An estimation based on the results of two population based studies. *Epilepsy Res* 1994; 18: 249–260.

34 Hall, B., Martin, E. and Smithson, H. *Epilepsy: A General Practice Problem.* London: Royal College of General Practitioners,1997.

35 Chappell, B. Epilepsy: patient views on their condition and treatment. *Seizure* 1992; 1: 103–109.

36 Dawkins, J.L., Crawford, P.M. and Stammers, T.G. Epilepsy: a general practice study of knowledge and attitudes among sufferers and non-sufferers. *Br J Gen Pract* 1993; 43: 453–457.

37 Jain, P., Patterson, V.H. and Morrow, J.I. What people with epilepsy want from a hospital clinic. *Seizure* 1993; 2: 75–78.

38 Jacoby, A. *Quality of Life and Care in Epilepsy*. Royal Society of Medicine Round Table Series No. 31, 1993: 66–73.

39 Freeman, G.K. and Richards, S.C. Personal continuity and the care of epilepsy in general practice. *Br J Gen Pract* 1994; 44: 395–399.

40 Chadwick, D. Seizures and epilepsy in adults. In: Laidlaw, J., Richens, A. and Chadwick, D. (eds) *A Textbook of Epilepsy*. Edinburgh: Churchill Livingstone, 1993: 165–204.

41 Hauser, W.A. and Kurland, L.T. The epidemiology of epilepsy in Rochester Minnesota 1935 through 1967. *Epilepsia* 1975; 16: 1–66.

42 Goodridge, D.M.G. and Shorvon, S.D. Epileptic seizures in a population of 6000. *Br Med J* 1983; 287: 641–647.

43 Rogers, D. and Taylor, M.P. *Don't Fit in Front of your Workmates—Living with Epilepsy in Doncaster*. Doncaster Medical Audit Advisory Group, Doncaster Health, 1996.

44 Kirby, S. and Sadler, R.M. Injury and death as a result of seizures. *Epilepsia* 1995; 36: 25–28.

45 Commission on Classification and Terminology of the International League against Epilepsy. Proposal for revised clinical and electroencephalographic classification of epileptic seizures. *Epilepsia* 1981; 22: 489–501.

46 Commission on Classification and Terminology of the International League against Epilepsy. Proposal for revised classification of epilepsies and epileptic syndromes. *Epilepsia* 1989; 30: 389–399.

47 Betts, T.A. and Boden, T. Pseudoseizures (non-epileptic attack disorder). In: M. Trimble (ed.) *Women and Epilepsy*. New York: John Wiley & Sons, 1991: 243–258.

48 Appleton, R., Baker, G., Chadwick, D. and Smith, D. *Epilepsy*, 3rd edn. London: Martin Dunitz, 1994.

49 Campbell-McBride, P. At the cutting edge. *Epilepsy Today*. March 1999: 8–10.

50 Walton, N. VNS: the Bristol experience. *Epilepsy Today*. March 2000: 8–10.

51 Strong, V., Brown, S.W. and Walker, R. Seizure alert dogs—fact or fiction? *Seizure* 1999; 8: 62–65.

52 Shorvon, S. *Handbook of Epilepsy Treatment*. Oxford: Blackwell Science, 2000.

53 Isojarvi, J.I.T., Laatikainen, T.J., Pakarinen, A.J., Juuteunen, K.T. and Myllyla, V.V. Polycystic ovaries and hyperandrogenism in women taking valproate for epilepsy. *N Engl Med J* 1993; 329: 1383–1388.

54 Wild, J.M., Martinez, C., Reinshagen, G. and Harding, G.F.A. Characteristics of a unique visual field defect attributed to vigabatrin. *Epilepsia* 1999; 40: 1784–1794.

55 Hoechst Marion Roussel. 'Important information on pharmacovigilance.' Hoechst, 27 August 1999.

56 Appleton, R.E. Guideline for prescribing vigabatrin in children has been revised. *Br Med J* 2000; 320: 1404–1405.

57 Ross, E.M., Peckham, C.S., West, P.B. and Butler, N.R. Epilepsy in childhood: findings from the National Child Development study. *Br Med J* 1980; 280: 207–210.

58 Crawford, P., Appleton, R., Betts, T., Duncan, J., Guthrie, E. and Morrow, J. Best practice guidelines for the management of women with epilepsy. *Seizure* 1999; 8: 201–217.

59 Crawford, C. Epilepsy in pregnancy (editorial). *Seizure* 1993; 2: 87–90.

60 Martin, G. People with learning disabilities: where do we go from here? *Br J Gen Pract* Sept 1999: 751.

61 Branford, D., Bhaumik, S. and Duncan, F. Epilepsy in adults with learning disabilities. *Seizure* 1998; 7: 473–477.

62 Kerr, M. Epilepsy in patients with learning disability. In: *Aspects of Epilepsy.* LibraPharm 1996; 3: 1–6.

63 Kerr, M. and Todd, S. *Caring Together in Epilepsy.* Cardiff: The Welsh Centre for Learning Disabilities.

64 Luhdorf, K., Jenson, L.K. and Plesner, A.M. Epilepsy in the elderly: incidence, social function, and disability. *Epilepsia* 1986; 27: 135–141.

65 Loiseau, J., Loiseau, P., Duche, B., Guyot, M., Dartigues, J.F. and Aublot, B. A survey of epileptic disorders in southwest France: seizures in elderly patients. *Ann Neurol* 1990; 27: 232–237.

66 Morrow, J. An assessment of an epilepsy clinic. In: Chadwick, D. (ed.) *Quality of Life and Quality of Care in Epilepsy.* London: Royal Society of Medicine, 1990: 96–105.

67 Scheepers, B., Pickles, C., Clough, P. and Harding, S. *The CARE Project—An Interim Report for the Department of Health.* London: Department of Health, 1997.

68 Scheepers, B. Epilepsy—Improving Care in the Community. *The National Association of Primary Care Official Review.* National Association of Primary Care, 1999.

69 Ridsdale, L., Robins, D., Cryer, C. *et al.* Feasibility and effects of nurse run clinics for patients with epilepsy in general practice: randomised controlled trial. *Br Med J* 1997; 314: 120–122.

70 Mills, N., Bachman, M.O., Harvey, I., Hine, I. and McGowan, M. Effect of a primary-care-based epilepsy specialist nurse service on quality of care from the patients' perspective: quasi-experimental evaluation. *Seizure* 1999; 8: 1–7.

Recommended further reading

Chadwick, D. and Usiskin, S. *Living with Epilepsy.* London: Macdonald Optima, 1992. [Written by a doctor and a patient and intended for patients and families, it is nevertheless a useful book for doctors and nurses, providing a simple and yet full account of epilepsy and its impact on patients and families.]

Oxley, J. and Smith, J. *The Epilepsy Reference Book.* London: Faber & Faber, 1991. [A source of questions and answers for patients, but also useful for health care workers.]

Appleton, R., Baker, G., Chadwick, D. and Smith, D. *Epilepsy.* London: Martin Dunitz, 1994. [A concise yet comprehensive clinically orientated book, mainly of use to junior hospital staff. Weak on the social aspects of epilepsy, but a very useful source of facts.]

Porter, R.J. *Epilepsy: 100 Elementary Principles*. London: W.B. Saunders, 1989. [A unique, fascinating and readable book. Full of practical wisdom presented in an unusual way which brings the management of patients with epilepsy to life.]

Laidlaw, J., Richens, A. and Chadwick, D. (eds) *A Textbook of Epilepsy*, 5th edn. Edinburgh: Churchill Livingstone, 1998. [A comprehensive textbook. It is authoritative and academic, mainly of value to specialists, but a useful source of reference for the rest of us.]

Shorvon, S. *Handbook of Epilepsy Treatment*. Oxford: Blackwell Science Ltd, 2000. [An up-to-date, clearly written source of information on treatment, especially on the application of the latest anti-epileptic drugs.]

Chappell, B. and Crawford, P. *Epilepsy at your Fingertips*. London: Class Publishing. 1999. [Contains useful practical information and tactics for dealing with problems including employment.]

Index

Page numbers in *italic* refer to figures or tables.

absence seizures 116
acetazolamide (Diamox) 95
  drug profile 83
acute symptomatic seizures 13
add-on drugs
  anti-epileptic drugs 50
  profiles 76–81
addiction, anti-epileptic drugs 134
advice
  adolescence 94
  elderly patients 105–6
  families 92–4, 109
  lifestyle implications 114
AED *see* anti-epileptic drugs
aetiology 13–14
age distribution (projected), Doncaster
    sample population *151*
age of onset 15
alarm systems 146
alcohol
  acute symptomatic seizures 13
  anti-epileptic drugs 135
  seizures 129–30
alternative therapies 137
An Epilepsy Needs Document
  seizure frequencies 16
  UK epilepsy services 6
anti-epileptic drugs (AED)
  carbamazepine metabolism 69
  childhood regimens *90*
  choice 49–53
  elderly patients 106–7
  knowledge 47–8
  learning disabilities 100–1
  over-the-counter medicines 135
  regimens 121–2
  treatment review 133
  treatment withdrawal 132

appointments 180–2
aromatherapy 67
assessment centres 169
atonic attacks 27
Attendance Allowance 144
audits
  care evaluation 7
  Community Awareness and Resources
      for Epilepsy project 160
  Doncaster Epilepsy Service 148
  general practice 172–6
  outpatients 183 185
automatisms 26

babies 99
behavioural therapy 66
benign partial epilepsies 88–9
benzodiazepines
  addiction 134
  side effects 81
biofeedback therapy 66
blood tests, frequency 135
books, patient information 171
brain damage, status epilepticus 124
brief flexion 25
British Epilepsy Association 167
bronchodilators 13

carbamazepine (Tegretol)
  drug profile 68–70
  introduction 3
  liver metabolism 48
  partial seizures 51
care plans 63
  general practices 155
  patients 55
CARE project *see* Community Awareness
      and Resources for Epilepsy project
care structures *154*
case studies 29–32
  diagnosis 35–41

case studies (*continued*)
  misdiagnosis 46–7
  newly diagnosed patients 55–7
CAT scan *see* computed tomography
catamenial epilepsy, acetazolamide 95
Centre for Community Neurological
  Studies 170
cerebral tumours 104
cerebrovascular disease
  elderly patients 104
  epilepsy incidence 152
checklist approach *110*, 111–22
childhood absence epilepsy 27
children
  epileptic seizures 87–8
  initial investigations 181
  treatment withdrawal 63
  vs. adults 84–5
chronic epilepsy
  acute seizures 13
  neurosciences centres 183
  treatment alteration 59–62, *61*
  treatment review 47
Citizen's Advice Bureaus 141
classifications, modern imaging
  techniques 19
clinical nurse specialists 161–2
clinical services, benchmarks 178
Clinical Standards Advisory Group
  (CSAG) 10
clobazam (Frisium)
  catamenial epilepsy 95
  drug profile 80–1
clonazepam (Rivotril) 81
clonic phase 25
Co-proxamol (dextropropoxyphene) 70
Community Awareness and Resources for
  Epilepsy project (CARE project) 160
community learning disability/learning
  disability epilepsy specialist nurses,
  roles 164–6
complex partial seizures (psychomotor
  epilepsy/temporal lobe epilepsy) 23
computed tomography (CT)
  children 86
  diagnosis 43
  initial investigations 180
  process 126–7
computer screens, photosensitive epilepsy
  114, 139
contraception
  anti-epileptic drugs 52, 120, 136
  enzyme-inducing anti-epileptics 96

council tax benefit 144
counselling 35
'critical mass', effective services 152–3
CSAG *see* Clinical Standards Advisory
  Group
CT *see* computed tomography
cumulative incidence rates *15*

DDA *see* Disability Discrimination Act
definitions, epilepsy 12–13
dextropropoxyphene *see* Co-proxamol
diagnosis
  children 85–91
  elderly patients 104
  levels 20
  mentally disabled patients 100
  principles 35
  review 41–2
Diamox *see* acetazolamide
diazepam (Valium)
  administering 128
  benzodiazepines 81
  status epilepticus 62
diets, ketogenic 136
diffuse cerebral disorders 17
Disability Discrimination Act (DDA) 115
Disability Living Allowance
  components 143
  Orange Badges 145
Disability Working Allowance 144–5
Disabled Persons Railcard 145
disclosure, Driving and Vehicle Licensing
  Agency 117
discos, photosensitive epilepsy 139
district structures, epilepsy services 153–4
dogs, seizure detection 66
Doncaster Epilepsy Service, case study
  148–9
driving licences
  Driving and Vehicle Licensing Agency
  170
  regulations 137–8
driving regulations 117–18
Driving and Vehicle Licensing Agency
  (DVLA) 116, 170
drop *see* atonic attacks
drug-resistant epilepsy 125
drugs
  acute symptomatic seizures 13
  choice, seizure types *51–2*
  interactions 48–9
  regimens *54*, 133
  withdrawal 48

DVLA *see* Driving and Vehicle Licensing
    Agency

EEG tests
    electrodes 65
    epilepsy classification 42–3
    process 126
elderly patients 104–7
    Attendance Allowance 144
electroencephalography 86
Emeside *see* ethosuximide
emotional development 130
employment
    barred occupations 114–15
    Disability Discrimination Act 139
    Health and Safety at Work Act 138
Epanutin *see* phenytoin
epidemiology, epilepsy 14–17
Epilepsy Association of Scotland
    address 167–8
    checklist approach *111*
epilepsy colonies 4
epilepsy services
    addresses 169
    management objectives *153*
epilepsy syndromes
    classifications 27–9, *28*
    definition 19
Epilepsy Wales 168
Epilim *see* sodium valproate
erythromycin 70
ethosuximide (Emeside/Zarontin)
    absence seizures 52
    childhood absence epilepsy 27
    drug profile 81–2
exercise 129
extension, tonic–clonic seizures 25

febrile convulsions 120
febrile seizures 87
fertility 95
first aid 112–13
first-line drugs
    anti-epileptic drugs 49–50
    profiles 68–71
    seizure types *51*
foetal development 131
follow-ups, patients 182–3
Frisium *see* clobazam
Fundholding 10

gabapentin (Neurontin)
    children 91

drug profile 77
introduction 4
partial/secondarily generalized seizures
    50
Gabitril *see* tiagabine
gamma knife surgery 65
general practices
    existing case management *157*
    management 155–8
generalized seizures
    definition 12–13, 24–7
    less-common types 27
girls, drug choice 52
glass 121
grand mal *see* tonic–clonic seizures

hair regrowth, sodium valproate 71
half-life, carbamazepine 69
health and safety 121
holidays 141
home visits 162–3
hormone replacement therapy 136
hormones 131
hypoglycaemic drugs 13

identification bracelets 170
idiopathic epilepsies 27–8, 120
immunizations 120
Incapacity Benefit 142
Income Support 143
Industrial Injuries Disablement Benefit
    144
infants 85
information collection, audits 173–4
inheritance 120
insurance
    driving 117
    employers 115
    health 141
intracarotid amytal test (Wada test) 65
Irish Epilepsy Association, The 168
Isoniazid 13

Jackson, Dr H. 3
Jacksonian seizures *see* simple partial sei-
    zures
Job Seekers Allowance 142
Jones, L. 8–9
juvenile myoclonic epilepsy 28
    myoclonic jerks *29*

Keppra *see* levetiracetam
ketogenic diets 136

Lamictal *see* lamotrigine
lamotrigine (Lamictal)
 carbamazepine 69
 drug profile 73–4
 introduction 4
 partial/generalized seizures 50
 sodium valproate 52, 71
LEA *see* local education authorities
learning disabilities 18
 community nurse assessments 186–92
 epilepsy 100–3
levetiracetam (Keppra)
 add-on anti-epileptics 50
 drug profile 79–80
 introduction 4
 seizure types 52
lignocaine 13
litigation, anti-epileptic drugs 97
liver metabolism, anti-epileptic drugs 48
local education authorities (LEA),
  Statutory Assessment 116, 139
localization related epilepsies 29
Losec *see* omeprazole
Luminal *see* phenobarbitone

magnetic resonance imaging (MRI)
 children 86, 127
 diagnosis 19, 43
management, GP roles 10
memory, anti-epileptic drugs 127–8
memory tests, surgery 65
menopause 99
menstrual cycles 95
Mersey Region Epilepsy Association 168
midazolam
 benzodiazepines 81
 status epilepticus 62
misdiagnosis
 challenging therapy 46–7
 seizures 36
 special centre referrals 7
mortality rates
 Doncaster sample population 151
 epilepsy 124
 National General Practice Study of
  Epilepsy 17
MRI *see* magnetic resonance imaging
myoclonic seizures 27
Mysoline *see* phenobarbitone

National General Practice Study of
  Epilepsy (NGPSE) 17
National Health Service (NHS) 149

National Insurance contributions, Job
  Seekers Allowance 142
National Society for Epilepsy, The 168
NEAD *see* non-epileptic attack disorder
Neurontin *see* gabapentin
new cases, management *156*
New Testament, tonic-clonic seizure 1–2
NGPSE *see* National General Practice
  Study of Epilepsy
NHS *see* National Health Service
non-epileptic attack disorder (NEAD/
  pseudo-seizures/psychogenic
  seizures) 38–40
 vs. epileptic seizures *39*
non-epileptic attacks, children *86, 88, 89*
non-specialists, learning disabilities 103
Nootropil *see* piracetam
nurses
 home visits 162–3
 specialist 161–3, 164–5
 training 159–60, 169–70

oestrogen metabolism 49
oils 67
omeprazole (Losec) 70
oral contraceptive pills 49
Orange Badges, parking 145
outpatient services, purchasing 177–85
overprotection, children 93
oxcarbazepine (Trileptal)
 carbamazepine 69
 carbamazepine titration 72
 drug profile 71–3
 introduction 4
 liver metabolism 48

partial seizures 12–13
partial seizures (localization-related)
 secondarily generalized seizures *22, 23,
  24*
patients
 concerns 44
 learning disabilities 101–2
 newly diagnosed 46, 53–5
 numbers 7, 180–2
 questions 123–41
 review 58–59, 157–8
PCGs *see* Primary Care Groups
penicillin 13
pertussis immunization 120, 131
petit mal *see* primary generalized
  seizures; simple absence
phenobarbitone (Luminal/Prominal)

drug profile 75
introduction 3
liver metabolism 48
phenytoin (Epanutin)
drug profile 74–5
introduction 3
liver metabolism 48
sodium valproate 71
photosensitive epilepsy 114
piracetam (Nootropil)
drug profile 82–3
introduction 4
polytherapy, drug withdrawal 48
potassium bromide 3
practice nurses 163–4
preconceptual counselling 96–7
pregnancies
anti-epileptic drugs 53, 97–8, 131
malformations 96
prescriptions
brand vs. generic 55, 134
charges 132–3
prevalence, Doncaster sample population
150–1
Primary Care Groups (PCGs) 149
primary generalized seizures (idiopathic
generalized epilepsies)
neural activity 25
sodium valproate 51–2
primidone (Mysoline)
drug profile 75
see also phenobarbitone
Prominal see phenobarbitone
prognoses, seizure control 113
prognostic factors 17
pseudo-seizures see non-epileptic attack
disorder
psychogenic seizures see non-epileptic
attack disorder
psychomotor epilepsy see complex partial
seizures
psychotropic drugs 13
public transport 145

referrals 34
new patients 179
remission rates
prognosis 113
seizures 17
remote symptomatic epilepsy see chronic
epilepsy
Report of the Working Group on Services
for People with Epilepsy 5

research, general practice 8
residential centres 168–9
Rivotril see clonazepam

Sabril see vigabatrin
savings, Income Support 143
schools
children with epilepsy 169
gyms 140
seizures 139
second-line drugs
anti-epileptics 49–50, 71–5
seizure types 51
seizure aetiology vs. age of onset 14
seizure alert dogs 66
seizures
classifications
old terms 21–2
treatment 20
driving licenses 118
elderly patients 105–6
food/drink 129
main groups 12–13
patient information 112
precipitating factors 113–14
prevalence 16
remission rates 17
vs. behaviour 101–2
serum levels, anti-epileptic drugs 53–5
Services for Patients with Epilepsy,
Clinical Standards Advisory Group
10
Severe Disablement Allowance 144
sex
anti-epileptic drugs 130–1, 134
anxiety 125
sexuality, desire vs. arousal 119
siblings 93
side-effects, anti-epileptic drugs 48, 133–4
simple absence (petit mal) 26
simple partial seizures 22
smoking 140
Social Service Departments 145
sodium valproate (Epilim)
childhood absence epilepsy 27
children 91, 92
drug profile 70–1
introduction 3
special educational needs, local education
authority 139
specialist nurses
compliance 59
epilepsy 159

spina bifida
  carbamazepine 69
  sodium valproate 71
sport 118–19
sports 140
Statement of Special Educational Needs,
      local education authorities 116
status epilepticus, treatment 62
street drugs 140
strokes, elderly 152
sudden unexplained death in epilepsy
      (SUDEP) 17
surgery 136
  operation types 64
  work-up 64–5
syncope vs. epilepsy
  case study 36
  differences 37

Tegretol *see* carbamazepine
temporal lobe epilepsy *see* complex
      partial seizures
temporal lobes, menstrual irregularity
      130
therapeutic earnings 144
tiagabine (Gabitril)
  drug profile 79
  introduction 4
tolerance, anti-epileptic drugs 133
tonic seizures 27
tonic–clonic seizures 25, *26*
Topamax *see* topiramate
topiramate (Topamax)

children 91
drug profile 78
introduction 4
travelling, medication 140–1
treatment
  beginning 45, 46
  development 3–4
  newly diagnosed patients 53–5
  surgical 63–6
  withdrawal 62–3
tremor, tonic–clonic seizures 25
Trileptal *see* oxcarbazepine

vagal nerve stimulation 65–6
Valium *see* diazepam
videos, patients 171
vigabatrin (Sabril)
  children 91
  drug profile 76–7
  infantile spasms 50
Vit K1, pregnancy 98

Wada test *see* intracarotid amytal test
waiting lists, outpatients 179
warfarin metabolism 69
water, safety 121
welfare benefits 141
witnesses, diagnosis 156
women
  drug choice 52–3
  epilepsy 94–9

Zarontin *see* ethosuximide